PLACES I'VE TAKEN MY BODY

ALSO BY MOLLY MCCULLY BROWN

The Virginia State Colony for
Epileptics and Feebleminded

In the Field Between Us
(with Susannah Nevison)

PLACES I'VE TAKEN MY BODY

ESSAYS

MOLLY MCCULLY BROWN

A KAREN & MICHAEL BRAZILLER BOOK
PERSEA BOOKS / NEW YORK

Persea Books, Inc.
90 Broad Street
New York, New York 10004

Library of Congress Cataloging-in-Publication Data

Names: Brown, Molly McCully, 1991– author.
Title: Places I've taken my body : essays / Molly McCully Brown.
Description: New York, New York : Persea Books, [2020] | Summary: "In seventeen intimate essays, poet Molly McCully Brown explores living within and beyond the limits of a body-in her case, one shaped since birth by cerebral palsy, a permanent and often painful movement disorder. In spite of-indeed, in response to-physical constraints, Brown leads a peripatetic life: the essays comprise a vivid travelogue set throughout the United States and Europe, ranging from the rural American South of her childhood to the cobblestoned streets of Bologna, Italy. Moving between these locales and others, Brown constellates the subjects that define her inside and out: a disabled and conspicuous body, a religious conversion, a missing twin, a life in poetry. As she does, she depicts vividly for us not only her own life but a striking array of sites and topics, among them Mary Shelley's Frankenstein and the world's oldest anatomical theater, the American Eugenics movement, and Jerry Falwell's Liberty University. Throughout, Brown offers us the gift of her exquisite sentences, woven together in consideration, always, of what it means to be human-flawed, potent, feeling"— Provided by publisher.
Identifiers: LCCN 2019044336 (print) | LCCN 2019044337 (ebook) | ISBN 9780892555130 (cloth) | ISBN 9780892555154 (epub)
Subjects: LCSH: Brown, Molly McCully, 1991—Travel. | Brown, Molly McCully, 1991—Religion. | Women poets, American—21st century—Biography. | Cerebral palsied—United States—Biography. | Lone twins—United States—Psychology.
Classification: LCC PS3602.R722354 P53 2020 (print) | LCC PS3602.R722354 (ebook) | DDC 818/.603 [B]—dc23
LC record available at https://lccn.loc.gov/2019044336
LC ebook record available at https://lccn.loc.gov/2019044337

Book design and composition by Rita Lascaro
Typeset in Carat
Manufactured in the United States of America. Printed on acid-free paper.

First Edition

For my family, in all its iterations,
And for Susannah, who made this feel possible.

CONTENTS

PLACES I'VE TAKEN MY BODY

Muscle Memory

For the last six months or so, whenever I've moved suddenly—stood up out of a chair, bent down to get my laundry from the machine, sneezed too hard in line at the convenience store up the block from my apartment—my back has spasmed, as if someone's making a quick, hard fist around my spine and squeezing. At first, it was just a twinge, enough to startle me. These days, it knocks me off balance if I don't brace for it first. And so I stretch more, and I stand and count to three before I step, or carry my coffee cup away from the table, or crouch down to put the dishes in the cabinet. I turn off the fan in the bedroom while I sleep, though it's May in Mississippi and already eighty degrees. Better to wake up sweating than knotted and tremoring from some little chill.

They're tiny, these adaptations. I suspect it took me months to notice I was making them. My life is built to flex unconsciously around new pain. I couldn't even tell you what I used to do with the small space the spasms fill. This version of my life erases the last one, like a tape someone's recorded over. Already, my memories begin reworking themselves to admit the spasms' brief delay: two seconds tacked on to the end of everything, a touch more hurt.

I haven't been to see a doctor because the change has so far been manageable. Because another dose of ibuprofen, a little less energy, and a slightly stronger ache to cope with isn't going to hurt me, really. I haven't been to see a doctor because I'm finishing graduate school and caught in the bureaucracy of going: no permanent address, shifting health insurance, too much in flux, and way too much to do.

I haven't seen a doctor because I haven't had a steady orthopedist since I outgrew the pediatric one I saw until I was eighteen. They treat cerebral palsy aggressively when you're young, your brain and body at the height of their plasticity. There's money to be spent on research and the promise of real progress to be made. They split your nerves, lengthen your tendons, splint your legs and map your changing gait with digital sensors that form points of light on the computer screen to indicate your muscles and your joints. This little constellation-self staggers the same blank orbit each year, getting taller. And then your body and brain have been reshaped as radically as medicine will currently allow, and you're just who you are and there are the ensuing years to manage on your own.

I haven't seen a doctor because my body has been mostly this version of itself for more than a decade now, and they've been mostly good years; I know the map of who I am and how I move by instinct, like home. I haven't seen a doctor because they'll want to alter something major, or they'll tell me that there's nothing to be done, that this is just my body's slow erosion asserting itself beyond ignoring, and either way there'll be a new geography to reckon with. I haven't seen a doctor because I am afraid. I haven't seen a doctor because there's too much to be said for feeling familiar to yourself. This is all the truth.

Another truth: before I knew this body, I knew another, nimbler one.

My very first body, the one untouched by major surgical intervention, exists only before my memory. For all intents and purposes, I wake into the world at the moment of its refashioning. My first clear recollection at four years old: somebody's hand hovering over my face, the weird cage of the gas mask, a dense, false butterscotch mingled with the drug. No memory, of course, of what they did while I was under; they give you something to induce forgetting. But the body I woke up with, I know it served me well for years.

I know the surgeons clipped select nerves in my spinal cord, and thereby cut off at the pass the bulk of my brain's bad commands to my muscles to contract beyond functionality or comfort. I know enough to know that I was born again then, in a looser shape, the one I first recognized as mine.

*

And it's in *that* body that I spent my childhood. I moved stutteringly around my grade-school classrooms. I wore opaque, plastic leg braces that stopped at my calves and sneakers two sizes too big for my real feet that made me look like a girl playing dress-up as a circus clown. I never played tag or kickball. But I could slowly climb the stairs to the splintering wooden castle and go down the slide. I could haul myself up to the monkey bars and swing along them just long enough to fall and split my lip like children do. The cut there bled a bright and normal red that made my mother woozy while they stitched it up. There isn't any scar.

And once, I could hop. I remember, because when I finally learned in the basement of the Baptist hospital—straining to reach a tennis ball the physical therapist held on a stick above my head—my father bought an ice-cream cake from Dairy Queen, all chemical soft-serve sweet, and we had a little party in the brightness of our farmhouse kitchen. I did it on command: two inches, maybe, off the ground. I know it happened, but that little space below my feet feels like a fiction now, held up against the relentless fact of gravity.

My family took a trip to Europe when I was nine years old. My parents, on sabbatical from college teaching jobs, swapped houses with a Spanish novelist and his wife, and for months we walked on the beaches of the Mediterranean and through the rocky outcrops to the north where Spain borders France. I remember flashes of those months with wild specificity: the garden of blooming cacti outside our little terracotta villa; playing rummy with my sister in the heat, on the flat roof, while someone blared a bizarre pop song about a cockroach from the bad speakers of the radio next door. I can see the winding maze of the nighttime street markets, full of Pokémon knockoffs and hand-painted bowls, humming with twinkle-lights and half-drunk bodies; the huge, cool steps of all the old churches turned into hotels; the wooden rollercoaster edging out toward the cliff face; that strange, spindly castle that wound up and up and up until you climbed its stairs and passed right through the clouds and to the other side.

In pictures, I'm standing at the top of the castle landing, in the shadow of the cathedral doors, on the wide, white wash of some uninterrupted beach. I walked and climbed through cities centuries too old for elevators, and across streets paved in big, uneven cobblestones. I threaded myself through a little monastery door and up a flight of improvised stone stairs into a walled garden, wrapped up in green. I can't remember getting there: not crossing the hill to the church grounds, not standing waiting for the door to give, not moving through the airy halls or up the stairs. If I try to picture it now, I can only envision myself up to the threshold. My memory of myself pauses and waits, but there isn't enough left of that balance or energy even for the purposes of recollection. I can imagine myself walking up through the monastery only in the same sense I can imagine that I flew.

You never recall what you do by instinct and, while my parents paused at every turn to say *remember this*, they meant the huge embroidered tapestries, the deep ring of the chapel bell, the way the air smelled hot but also dense with moss that wasn't there. No one knew enough to warn me that the body I had then would go to myth in my mind much faster than any of the rest of it.

It's probably natural to recall change, the moment that one season shifts into another, and so it's not surprising that I remember my early body most strongly in the time just before it didn't exist anymore. When I tell the story, I compress and exaggerate for narrative's sake, say: *Basically, I hit puberty and then woke up one morning and mostly couldn't walk.* This isn't strictly true, of course. It happened more slowly than all that, but quickly enough to worry us all and baffle my doctors. My joint pain and balance got rapidly worse, and I started moving through our house by leaning heavily on one piece of furniture and then the next—couch, chair, end table, counter—my eyes watering with the effort.

In my memory, though, my early body's going has a single, undeniable beginning, just before my rapid decline in mobility: one so storybook that if I hadn't lived it, I would swear I made it up.

The house where I was raised, on a college campus in the mountains of nowhere Virginia, backed up on a long series of rolling fields. When I was very young, they'd been cow pastures, but for most of my life they were bucolic, uninhabited country, mowed for sweet, colossal bales of hay. My younger brother and I spent whole afternoons out there, picking our way through the pasture with other faculty kids down to the furrow of a creek that ran below the first rusted hill. I'd already developed, by then, a taste for being alone, and I would often break off from the group and make my way down through the brambles into one of the little red clay hollows cut into the side of the hill. My favorite was a thicket, heavy with honeysuckle, with a gnarled old oak tree rising up out of the center. It was the perfect tree for climbing: huge and covered with footholds. In my old body, I could reach its middle branches clumsily and settle myself steady in the crook of them: look up and out. I don't remember the climbing, but I remember the sky. I passed hours like that.

One afternoon I made my way out to the tree. I suspect the walk was already becoming hard, although I don't recall that part, only that, when I arrived, I couldn't get my foot to the first branch, couldn't lift my leg quite high enough or force my toe to catch. I sweated and wept, and I tried so long my parents came out hunting for me, knowing where I'd gone. My mother, crying too, and deeply patient, sent my father back to the house for a step stool, which he carried out over the long grass. But even with that help I couldn't make it. Together, they could lift me up, but there was no more climbing. My father carried me, heavy and wailing way too hard for nearly eleven, back to the house.

A year or so later, in the thick of the physical disintegration that day at the climbing tree had heralded, I got my period in the bathroom of my grandmother's house. My mother swore loudly from the other side of the door when I told her, *Shit! Oh no!* She banged in, eyes watering, touching me roughly, not meeting my gaze. I know, now, that her roughness came from grief and terror. I was growing up into a perplexing and unstable body that she had no idea how to help me manage. There wasn't any road map. I hurt like hell. We had no idea what was coming. We growled at each other as my old body dimmed in the distance, both much too good at converting sadness and fear into fury. For a day we didn't talk. It took me years to learn enough to really forgive her.

The effects of spasticity wear away at your joints, but cerebral palsy isn't degenerative. The neurological damage is static and consistent, and no one knew what to make of my rapid decline in mobility, my rapid increase in pain. For more than a year, we shuttled back and forth between my orthopedist and a neurologist. After several MRIs, I got used to the loud, hollow clanking, the narrow press of the imaging tube. My parents and I people-watched in waiting rooms and laughed behind our hands at some of what we overheard. One chair over, an old woman answered a questionnaire. *Have you had any surgery in the past eight weeks?* the nurse inquired. *Not that I'm aware of,* the woman sang back loudly, brightly. It's funny at first blush: Of course you'd know if you'd had surgery! But now I think how quickly the forgetting happens, one body replaced so utterly by another. Who can trust what happened in that other shape?

There was never any change in my brain scans or my spinal cord, never any tumor or other explanation. Once, in the parking lot, after another identical set of images, I wept all of sudden. I had a wheelchair by then—not the little, black, sporty one I'd come to use just a few months later, but one of those huge hospital folding numbers, a stopgap measure to cope with the new reality.

My mother bent down to meet my eyes: *You know you're not sick, right?* she said. *You're not sick.* But that wasn't why I was crying. I hadn't really ever been afraid of that, though I suspect that she might have been. I could tell that whatever was happening was just the world of me reshaping. I missed my old margins, missed knowing myself. I didn't know yet that soon I'd also lose the memory of how I used to move.

The explanation we finally settled on was everybody's best hypothesis: When I grew and gained weight in the quick, clumsy way you do in adolescence, my muscles, without the help of several neural pathways severed in that early experimental spinal surgery, couldn't naturally gain the necessary strength to keep pace with the rest of me. As my spasticity got worse, so did my balance, and my joints bore much more weight, which made my walking even tighter, more labored, and unstable: this bad, invisible cycle repeating quickly as a synapse fires, or fails to.

The surgery was still a good idea, they think. It's the standard of care now for many young children with CP. Without that initial loosening, I wouldn't have had all those good, relatively mobile years, and who knows what body I would be in now. But combating its byproducts meant that, for most of junior high, I went to school only part time while I spent half my day in physical therapy or at the gym. It meant having my tendons lengthened yet again, and stints in plaster casts and full-length braces that locked my legs in place with a huge metal hinge. I wore parachute pants to cover them up, and even bigger sneakers. All of it hurt with a kind of constancy that set my teeth perpetually on edge. My body's replacement was violent; I bled when I shed my skin.

Within a few years, though, I had mostly settled back down into this new body, made my home there. I could walk, a little, though it still hurt some. I was familiar to myself again and busy and distracted by all the things I wanted from the world. I left home and moved every few years, hungry to test out my new shape in new, clear territory.

I won't say I still miss walking like I used to. I don't remember it well enough to grieve, except in the abstract.

Truthfully, I hadn't realized how much motion I'd lost to forgetting until I tried to remember: standing painlessly, playing in a riverbed, ascending a staircase untouched, leaving the ground for an instant in a jump, climbing up a tree to get closer to the sky. I'm sorry that I can't conjure memory of any of that, that I can't bring up a map of the girl who did those things or remember what it was like to have her skin. I don't recall inhabiting her body until the point at which it started breaking.

And maybe this is just some strange, exaggerated version of what it means to age: huge sections of our lives lost to the way memory buckles and muddies and fades, the versions of ourselves we couldn't find our way back toward if we tried. But as I lose the girl I once was to forgetting, she takes with her a whole collection of places, her particular windows on the world. She saw things I never will.

I'm about to go to Europe again, for the first time since that childhood trip. I'm scheduled for a six-week artist's residency that stretches out before me like a spotlight on the lucky fact of my life. This time I won't walk anywhere. To

PLACES I'VE TAKEN MY BODY

prepare, I spend hours on the phone confirming doorway widths to be sure my wheelchair will fit. I inquire about elevator functions and the height of bathtub lips. I cross whole Italian cities off my list because their streets are only stairs and cobblestones. I surprise myself by being grateful that I'm traveling to a different country this time around. I don't want to go back to that Spanish monastery to find that I can't get inside. It's enough to be trapped at the thresholds of my memories. I don't think I could bear stalling at a real threshold: *Once, you could be here.* Every inch I can no longer walk, the world shrinks just a little, the edges of the map curl in. There are places I will never go. There are places I will never go again.

I told you that after I made a home in my new body, I was hungry for new places. I grew devoted to the act of going, just to prove I could. Every eighteen months or so I'd train my eyes on some distant city and think *there,* and muscle my way into a different life. *Now I've done it,* I'd think. *I've been here. I've seen it.* New England buried in thick drifts of snow. The sharp, apocalyptic gorgeousness of Northern California's cliffs. West Texas scrub, and all of Austin's reluctant, trendy glitz. And on again from there, to other southern towns and different kinds of weather. Each time I left a whole life behind without really bothering to glance in the rearview mirror, peeling away hurried and messy and loud. Only now does it occur to me that I was rushing so rapidly, not just toward the promise of being somewhere new, but away from the old place before it became too familiar. I never wanted to know anywhere well enough or long enough to notice when I lost pieces of it to my body's slow degeneration, when I couldn't make my way into certain spaces anymore. I needed to leave a place before a place left me.

My parents still live on the same college campus where I was raised, but about a year ago they moved into a different house, away from the fields. I went back to Virginia to help prepare for the move, and the morning before they left our house for good, I stood out at the lip of the field and looked toward the place I knew my climbing tree was hidden. I hadn't been out there in more than a decade, and in the intervening years they'd stopped mowing the hills regularly. The summer grass was high and thick and swaying in the hot wind, grown nearly up to my eyeline. Really, that whole space was memory in almost every sense now. Most of what I could see was the sky over where I once climbed. Bigger, I thought, from lower down. I could only stand there for a minute. Quickly my knees began to buckle, and I had to stumble back toward the house.

I'm trying to get better at not stealing places from myself too early, at staying long enough to commit whole swaths of them to real, true memory and to be grateful for them.

Underneath my skin, I know my body is remaking itself again in some slower but significant way. This is always happening, quietly. Already, the past is rewiring itself. My memory of who I am pauses at another threshold. I can't keep her, but I hope she stays familiar to me. I would like to stay on nodding terms with who and where I've been. I would like to remember this, please: standing almost straight up at the mirror, aching just a little, my own hands working sure and steady in my hair.

IN SMOKE AND EXHAUSTION

In Bologna, seemingly everyone smokes. The old man with one bad hand drinking a giant piña colada asks the waitress to light his cigarette, and when she bends to spark her lighter near the tip, the whole thing disappears behind the flame, and for a second I can only see the fire and her fingers, then the small world of his mouth. I watch a teenage girl outside the same café spinning a cigarette, which she looks way too young to have purchased, while she sips a Coke. A boy across the table laughs at something she's just said. That night, a woman smokes alone between bites of lasagna. She looks at her phone, talks with the waiter, pulls a blazer over her shoulders as the night gets cooler. She lights more cigarettes through red wine, then coffee, then the walk off to wherever it is she's going. She isn't beautiful, but she has elegant hands. Fingernails like pale and perfect boats.

Everywhere, the tarry smell reminds me of a headache. The bar down the block from the apartment where I'm staying is called *Coffee and Cigarettes*, rare English lit up in a neon sign. There's a whole wall of foil packs behind the counter:

black, and red, and blues like bodies of water with different depths. I have no appetite at all, and every time I pass the door I almost buy a pack, the impulse to whittle myself away to nothing an old cliché, one I thought I'd lost the reflex for. Instead, I drink four espressos in an hour and get empty-stomach-tipsy on one strong cocktail—but not more than one, because I am afraid of getting lost or falling down. The flimsy, combined buzz is almost enough that I feel briefly bodiless as long as I don't try to get up from the table. I try not to get up from the table for as long as I can.

I'm here a year. And by *here* maybe I mean this city, but probably I just mean *not America,* mean *on the road.* I'm on a fellowship that pays me for being gone. One American poet a year is funded just to spend that time abroad, to write back from a foreign place. The list of previous winners is a list of heroes. The time is a gift. Right now, I am spending it getting shallowly drunk at a wrought iron table and wondering whether the disappearance of my hunger is due more to fear, or physical pain, fatigue, or anger at my broken and breakable body, and if an absence can be equal parts that many things.

A few weeks in, I'm discovering that being abroad in a wheelchair engenders an intense kind of myopia that feels both necessary and dangerous: this sense that I have to pay so much attention to my own body, to the ground right in front of me, to the impending set of stairs, that I never really see anything at all except the shattered blue beer bottle I almost run over, the stray cobblestone I spot just before it pitches me out of the wheelchair and into the busy street, the sign for an elevator that leads nowhere except back to where I began. I pass again and again by an extraordinary view of a peach-colored church deepening in sunset while looking for a ramp into Bologna's public library. Circle it five or six times before I even notice. I have to force myself to keep a list of things I see beyond my body: a huge chocolate lab passed out on the laundromat floor; graffiti outside my apartment door that reads *eat the rich*; all the smoking citizens, their mouths and hands. Otherwise I will have thought only about my own hands, darkening with grime from the city street, and about tracking the pulse of pain in my lower back for a whole afternoon, a day, a week. I worry that, because my body goes with me everywhere, it won't matter how far I travel, that I'll still just be telling its same small story over and over again. That this is all wasted on me.

One evening, I call my parents and, discussing my plans for the year, my mother asks if my ambition to learn Italian is lessening. I laugh a little meanly, because the notion that I might speak any language at all beyond the language of my body feels suddenly absurd. And then, because she means the question so tenderly and with such worry, I bite the laughter back, just say, *We'll see.*

I was here two days before I got a flat wheelchair tire, leaving me stranded, frightened, and immobilized. And—in my better moments since then—I've been looking for places where silence means *peace* and not *loneliness,* because I've spent enough time traveling alone to know that contemplative spaces can help combat fear and isolation. I discover a botanical garden a block from my apartment: canopies of trees, bright green and alive. But the paths through the whole thing are poured white gravel, pristine and impassible in the chair. I pause at the gate a little while, turn back to my apartment, go home and pull my body into bed.

I think that maybe I should go to Mass: the ritual the same in every language, a chance to practice gratitude and intentional stillness rather than paralysis. So, one Saturday, I go to explore churches, figuring I'll devote a whole day of preparation to my body's limits before Sunday's service. I stop at two, but they have big, gorgeous stone stairs outside every door that I can find, and the whole enterprise sours. All I want is to be able to come in and be swallowed by the motions of the crowd. Everything around me is beautiful. I can't make myself keep looking. Instead, I look again at my own body: *All of this is wasted on you.*

Across the ocean, my closest friend, Susannah, texts, *Please be gentle with yourself.* And, because I love her, I promise her I am. And I am trying to be. But I hate it. I feel utterly untender with myself. There are so many places that I want to be, but I can't take my body anywhere. But I must take my body everywhere.

Feeling guilty and exhausted, I keep rereading Rebecca Mead's essay "A New Citizen Decides to Leave the Tumult of Trump's America" in the *New Yorker*. She writes about choosing to move with her family back to England, where she was born, in the aftermath of the 2016 election. About deciding that they had to go, and about knowing she'll come back to America one day, knowing that she can.

I can't stop thinking about how she discusses the privilege of that choice, what it means to be able to migrate, to move about freely. Our government is increasingly xenophobic and isolationist. At the United States' southern border, hundreds of children are separated from their parents. Families torn apart often just because they dared to *ask* for the privilege of motion, dared to ask to come in where they might be safe, where they might find opportunity.

It's a loaded and remarkable moment to have been granted, by virtue of my citizenship, my education, and my art, the freedom and resources to go practically anywhere, just to see it, just to expand my own experience of the world. A remarkable time to have been told: *Go to every great monument. Every far-flung city. Go to holy sites and hidden villages. Go someplace where you don't know the language to ask any of your questions. Learn it. Go live a life somewhere entirely unfamiliar.* In my usual life, I'm a teacher as well as a writer, and I always tell my students that one of the most powerful and important things they can do is to be invested in the complexity and value of an existence that looks nothing like their own, of places utterly unlike their homes. This fellowship makes that my only job for an entire year, and I keep stalling out at thresholds: aching, impeded, and lonely, reduced to studying the cuts on my own legs.

A little while ago, I published an essay which included a description of the difficulty of attending cocktail parties if you can't really stand. In the online comments section, one reader posted a response, the gist of which was, *Why the hell would you ever go to a party if you know it's just going to hurt and you can't really do it?* At the time, I laughed. But now I keep thinking about it.

Why the hell would you ever go someplace you know that you can't really be?

All of this is wasted on you.

I write this essay today largely because I am too sore and tired to muster up the energy or the courage to leave the apartment. I worry that, at a moment when the freedom of motion across borders is in short supply, when global consciousness feels increasingly urgent, when so many artists are fighting for opportunities to keep themselves afloat, it is unforgivably selfish to have taken this opportunity away from someone who could make more expansive use of it; whose body wouldn't at every moment resist the remarkable permission for motion they'd been given; who could tell you, after weeks in this old and stunning city, about more than the hands of the people who smoke here: how they are beautiful, and moving, and then gone.

I chose this city to begin in partly because it's the one where men began to map the human body, the one where surgery was born. But all that I can catalog now are the ways it couldn't fix me. And now we've reached the limits of the present tense, because I cannot even tell you yet when I'll be hungry next, and the whole future is conditional, I hope there's something in these pages worth preserving. I hope I'll get more capable as things grow more familiar. I hope I'll manage not to waste this gift. I hope tomorrow I will make it up and out.

If You Are Permanently Lost

I never have any idea where I am. I lived my whole childhood in the purple foothills of the same five-square-mile town, and I still can't tell you whether you turn left or right on the single thruway to get to the grade school or the grocery store, or how to find the houses of any of my childhood friends. I can't tell you how to find the conspicuously modern angles of the apartment building in the small town in Mississippi where I lived for the three years in graduate school, or even easily direct you from my old house in Austin to the bright little bar where I wrote much of my first book. I never know how far I am from the airport or the highway. I can't read a map effectively, and even though it's less than half a mile from my current apartment in London, I couldn't get to the Thames without the artificial voice on my cellphone—set to an Australian accent so its omnipresence is less tiresome—calling out *turn left* every two hundred and fifty feet. Half the time, to remember which way is left, I have to imagine for an instant that I am picking up a pen.

Even on a much smaller scale, space makes no sense to me. I walk all the way around the perimeter of a room to reach a door that's immediately to my right, and I set my glass down half an inch from the edge of the table with such frequency that anyone who knows me well gets used to nudging it back again and again over the course of an evening in this small, choreographed two-step. As a girl, I put my shoes on the wrong feet so reliably that my parents directed me just to behave in defiance of my inclinations; if I thought a sneaker should go on one foot, put it on the other. This is still a strategy I use sometimes. If I'm certain an office is to the right out of the elevator, I go left down the hall. I'm almost always wrong about the layout of the world.

I come, after a while, to recognize landmarks—pale blue awning of the nearest dry cleaner, wrought iron railing along the railroad bridge, surprise of a green painted storefront among all the brick—which is how I learn, eventually, to navigate some frequent paths of travel, but no collection of spaces, no matter how habitually I move through them, ever knits into any kind of coherent map inside my head. I'll be wandering in the city convinced I'm miles away from anywhere I've ever been, and then turn a corner just to see the shapes of my own block rising up as if they've been transplanted, their familiarity more unsettling than encountering something new, proof I lack a homing instinct of any kind.

There's a neurological explanation for at least some of this. The ability to process information about distance, angles, and direction—to reason, essentially, about the physical expanse around you—is called spatial cognition, and the oxygen deprivation at birth that caused my cerebral palsy resulted in some injury to the neural structures that make this kind of reasoning possible, like a blown fuse in the wiring of my brain. Lights from down the hall provide a little glow, but the chamber is permanently dim.

More than that, though, it turns out that, in young children, spatial cognition begins to develop concurrently with what professionals term *independent locomotion*: the ability to get around under your own steam. Essentially, you gain the capacity to map the world as you begin to move intentionally through it, the brain wiring in sync with what the body does. I never wiggled or crawled effectively, my muscles too spastic and stiff, and I didn't learn to walk until I was four, which is too late for typical cognitive progress to occur. There's an allotted developmental window for the needed synchronicity to come to pass in, and if it doesn't, it's impossible to perfectly correct the disjunction. With attention, you can create some new neural pathways, alternate routes to comprehending space, but you can't retrace the steps you should have taken.

*

My terrible sense of direction is a long-running joke among family and friends, who know better than to trust my baseless assurances that I'm positive we're heading the right way this time, and for a long time my lack of spatial awareness mostly felt like an inconvenience, minor in comparison to my difficulty walking, or to chronic pain. But I've been thinking, lately, about home and navigation: what it means to be perennially dislocated, what it means when space, no matter how you try to fathom it, refuses to coalesce into a place you know.

*

Displaced from their breeding pools, marbled newts can only find their way back home when certain stars are visible; they spend whole days paused with their bellies pressed to the ground waiting for the sun to set, the clouds to clear. Homing pigeons' compass mechanisms rely on the sun, but when it's dark or clouded over, they can feel the earth's magnetic field. Iron particles collected in their beaks will always tug them toward true north. Honey bees navigate by polarized light, give directions to one another relative to the position of the sun. Bats and cave swiftlets and porpoises map intricate and perfect distances from echoes. And even mollusks, base and faceless, hold a topographic memory of the land, find their way via familiar contours: rises and gullies they remember how to fit inside. All these bodies that know home somewhere inside them.

It isn't at all that I don't get attached to landscapes: the exact color of the clay in the mountains where I was raised, part rust, part something redder; the miles and miles of cool blue flat driving through a Mississippi January morning; the wildness of California palm trees in the winter. There's a scent of Virginia magnolia, dusk-sweet and *too much*, that I can call up instantly, and my favorite sound is the particular loud, humid crack of a weirdly rainless Southern thunderstorm, come out of nowhere and then gone again. But you could put me down on the land I love most in the world, and I would still be lost inside it, the familiar made alien and unsteady by my inability to fuse its fragments to a whole.

I lived in six different cities and towns in the last ten years, and now two foreign countries in the last six months. Without really meaning to, I've made a life composed almost entirely of leaving and arrival, a life where it's reasonable to never know my way around. *I'm new*, I say, or, *I'm about to go*, or, *I don't live here, I'm just visiting.* I think, *This isn't my real life.*

At a medical library in London, I stand in front of a photographic print of the human brain and spinal column strung with nerves, magnified to many times its size. Hung there on the wall, huge and in black and white, it looks more than anything like a tangle of netting and driftwood and rope, like a raft someone assembled swiftly, in a panic, trying to survive a storm. I keep thinking of the last stanza of that Adrienne Rich poem "Song": *If I'm lonely / it's with the rowboat ice-fast on the shore / in the last red light of the year / that knows what it is, that knows it's neither / ice nor mud nor winter light / but wood, with a gift for burning.*

If there's any territory I should know well, it's the country of my own body. So much of my life has been devoted to attending to its margins and features: its tenuous center of gravity; the tense curl of my hamstrings and heel cords; the banks of calluses along the perimeter of my feet, hardened from years of walking on my toes with my feet listing stubbornly to one side; the thickets of scarring behind my knees and at my ankles, and the fading ridgeline where they sliced me open at the spine. I've had so many cartographers and architects: doctors' appointments and surgeries designed to know and map my body, alter its geography, to make it more habitable. It, at least, should be comprehensible: place instead of merely space.

But here there is a double alienation. Because the world refuses to grow knowable and navigable, because my brain cannot compose a cogent map, my body is rendered new to me each time I try to move through space. Each turned corner is an uncharted expanse I have no idea how I will traverse or respond to. And because my body itself has been reshaped so many times, both through the intentional, artificial manipulations of surgery, and by its own ongoing and present disintegration, I can't truly know or trust its geography either. The tectonic plates of who I am are always shifting. My friend

Susannah, another writer, has also had a great deal of surgery, her own profound erosions. This heavy grief, finally shared with another person, yielded a nearly instant bond between us. We both know there's no returning to the beginning, no knowing who you've always been, no going home again. But we also know that there's no staying where you are: that the moment that your body sutures together into a whole and steady place you know, something will give way and you'll be changed to mere parts again.

Sometimes I think I've made myself into a constant traveler as mechanism of defense. On a practical level, it's a bad strategy: to compound the permanent unfamiliarity my brain and body engender with still more newness, evolving practical obstacles in every unmappable place. But in another way, it makes a kind of sense. I'd rather be a stranger, transitory and alone, because of something I decided than as a consequence of something in me, some lack that proves again and again just what a damaged animal I am. Constant motion camouflages the extent to which I'm alien even to myself.

*

Again I return to Adrienne Rich's rowboat, beached on the cold shore. I think, *I don't know where or what I am.* But then, I consider how, in laying out a litany of what it knows it's not, Rich transfigures that rowboat again and again in the course of a single line: *boat* to *ice* to *mud* to *winter light* and finally to *wood*, raw material whose most miraculous property is its ability to burn, break down, to change. How it's a gift to alchemize to something else.

In the world of a poem, it's an advantage to be inescapably a stranger, an explorer. The task is so often to render the familiar changed and charged and new, or to chart a path through constantly evolving territory, thick with shifting shadows. The woman in Rich's "Song" drives continually onward, leaves behind *mile after mile / little towns she might have stopped / and lived and died in,* but the poem itself holds all those possible lives at once. The fragment is rendered its own small, self-contained place, its capacity for continual transformation a gift of metaphor, music, and line.

To work your way forward when you are permanently lost means, yes, to be exhausted and adrift, a stranger in a strange land. But, as a writer, it also means living in a state of endless discovery. The world unfurls itself anew each day with *dawn's first cold breath on the city.* You re-encounter what you are: lonely like a body with a gift for burning.

BENT BODY, LAMB

The last time I tell anyone I don't believe in God is the summer before ninth grade. My mother and I are lying in my parents' bed, still awake at 3 a.m. This is how we spend almost every night that July, because it is one hundred degrees even in the dark, and the casts on my legs extend from my toes all the way to my hips, and even with the maximum dosage of codeine and valium, I can't stop spasming long enough to sleep. My damaged brain sends one insistent command to the muscles in my legs: *contract, contract, contract.* They try to bend inside the plaster, and when they can't, they writhe. In the daylight, I sometimes joke that I'm possessed: a fucked-up marionette with jointless wooden legs. But at night, I don't feel like kidding. The backs of my legs are chafed and bleeding where the skin has been rubbed off, and there's only a moment or two of stillness between convulsions.

Lying there, in the sticky Virginia dark, I ask my mother whether or not she thinks there's a God. *I'm not sure*, she says. *I don't know.* The moon hangs large enough outside the bedroom window that I can see the outline of her tired, fine-boned face turn toward me in the bed, her hair wild on the pillow.

I am, I say, with stupid, feigned certainty engendered by adolescence and pain. *God isn't real.* I'm silent for half a beat and then, all of a sudden, I look at her and snarl, *This is all your fault.*

This is the cruelest possible thing I can say to my mother, who fears her body failed to keep my twin sister and me safe, delivering us into the world too early and too small, so that Frances died after less than thirty-six hours, and I emerged from the NICU with cerebral palsy, which renders my brain damaged and my body spastic, off-balance, and largely dependent on a wheelchair.

In fact, twins are at high risk for preterm birth and early rupture of their amniotic sacs. Frances and I were born at twenty-seven weeks and, between us, we weighed less than four pounds. My mother is blameless. But in her grief she doesn't feel that way, and I know that. I am lying when I tell her that I believe any of this is her fault. I'm also lying when I say I don't believe in God. She reaches out to touch my face and I yank my cheek away and turn my head. I can hear that she is crying.

*

The temptation is to say that having an identical twin who dies just after birth means living with the hieroglyph of loss carved into you from your earliest breath—but that's imprecise and a concession to melodrama. The truth is closer to this: You wake up in the morning just like everyone else wakes up in the morning; you resist the light coming in planks through the blinds; you pull your dress over your head. Usually, while doing this, you're thinking nothing or only that your feet are cold or that you wish you hadn't left your laundry unfolded in the basket overnight. Meanwhile, though, somewhere just outside you, this small, heated weight is hanging in the air. There is another heartbeat at the furthest edge of your hearing, and every glance of your body in your peripheral vision has the potential to feel suddenly stolen: You're looking at someone else's shoulder blade, even if it looks just like yours. This sense of another body—in yours—or barely beyond yours—or instead of yours—marks your life like a lighthouse lamp, waning and flaring in the distance.

I don't know who told me about Frances. She goes as far back as I can remember, and I know our origin story like a myth: the twinning of two identical girls in the safe dark of a mother's stomach, the violence with which they were torn from her, how they shuddered in the light. One girl clung to the messy new universe. The other abandoned her little body, streaming off in pursuit of another world. Each was a half of something.

*

What matters now is that the pale pink card that bears my birth announcement also bears the news of Frances's death. What matters is that my sister is a single, slim file in the back of a cabinet in our parents' house: two polaroids, a hospital bracelet, our ultrasound printouts, a footprint barely as wide as my thumb. What matters is that I know what her nose would look like, down to the small rise in the bridge, know how her voice would sound, but have never heard her say a word. What matters is that she would be a woman now.

Sometimes, lying in bed at night, I conjure the weight of her arm tossed over mine in the casual, intimate sleep of sisters, and I can almost swear that she's in bed beside me, the rise of her shoulder blade visible in a soft blue t-shirt, her face buried in the pillow, her legs and bare feet pulled in tight toward her body. Spastic, I still sleep curled up like I'm in the womb—the last place we were properly twinned. Sleeping, my tightened body makes a hollow built for her.

I am utterly certain some version of Frances persists somewhere. I feel her nearly constantly, and so I have to believe in some divinity, some life beyond this one I'm living. Even as I would like to throttle the God who killed her, I've always had to believe he's real. I have to believe that, somehow, there's an order to her early death and her brief life.

*

My family never went to church regularly when I was a child, but my parents sent me to Quaker school for a few years, and in college I start going quietly to Mass. The Cathedral is beautiful, and my father grew up Catholic, so I have some cultural affinity for the Church. It seems as natural a place as any to seek a present God. I sit in the back, and learn all the prayers, and never speak to anyone except in the moments immediately after the *Our Father*, when ritual dictates you turn and greet your neighbor. A few times I almost ask the priest about converting, stopping just short of actually having a conversation. In those years, I read a lot of John Milton, Gerard Manley Hopkins, and John Donne, and I carry Christian Wiman's deeply devotional poetry collection *Every Riven Thing* with me like a bible. I read King James scripture and dog-ear most of the pages in an anthology of stories about belief. I write almost exclusively about faith and its absence, and from all this I build and take apart a hundred Gods.

I dream the wild lover who took over Margery Kempe's body and made her wail, and the God Flannery O'Connor scratched on Parker's back. I wrestle with the personal, inflexible Christ promised by the billboards in the mountains at home in Virginia. I map the Lord onto a boy I adored as a young girl, one with a Carhartt jacket and a soft southern accent, a screwed-up family and eyes so clear, pale blue they sometimes looked like ice or air. I search out God in Virginia clay and the wood-heated house of my childhood neighbor, who played Christian television in the background all day and liked it when I read her Psalms out loud. I want a God who is rustic and resurrected and material, who will talk to me in the staticky silence I hear playing in my head all the time.

My senior year, I write an undergraduate thesis on *Paradise Lost.* I never miss a week of church. But my faith is a quiet, messy, and uncertain thing, largely secret and unspoken. I grew up twenty-five miles from Jerry Falwell's Baptist mega-church, in the heartland of what often feels like the worst religion has to offer: bigotry and prejudice, rabid anti-intellectualism, the inability to yield even a single hard-edged certainty up to kindness, questioning, or complication. I'm more than a little embarrassed by my desire for religion, which seems to me to conflict with both my progressive politics and my rational mind. So, while I've educated myself to be able to talk comfortably about the role of Christianity in literature, taken theology classes, and become a regular at Mass, I've continued to insist, in all my public posturing, on the kind of critical distance academia rewards. I learn to say, *I'm interested in religion* instead of *I'm desperate to feel close to God.* I explain, *I'm attracted to ritual* instead of *I know something transcendent happens when I pray a Hail Mary; I can actually feel the air heat up around me.* Sometimes I wear a little silver cross around my neck, but I make sure to keep it tucked underneath my sweater or my dress. I downplay its significance even to my college boyfriend, a sweet and logical Jewish agnostic.

It's just family jewelry, I say. *I like the history.*

I believe in some kind of God, I say, *but I'm not a Christian.*

*

In early August 2014, a new friend, Kate, and I are having dinner in my apartment in Oxford, Mississippi. I moved here just about a month ago to get a graduate degree in poetry, and she's the first real friend I've made. She's got one of those laughs you can tell emerges from a true place in the gut, and is prone to a rapid, slightly caustic banter I like because it matches mine. But, more than that, somehow I've already got the sense that I don't need to translate everything I say to her into some saner, more palatable form before it leaves my mouth; that, in fact, she understands a lot before I even vocalize it. She already knows about Frances, and now we're trading longer, messy backstories over risotto in that underwater light that marks a southern summer evening. *I care a lot about God,* I tell her, which is the truest thing I know how to say about it.

A week or two later, we're sitting at St. John the Evangelist, the Catholic church in Oxford. I marvel at how, even after a couple of years away from Mass, the routine feels intimately familiar. I make the sign of the cross, touching my forehead, then the shallow at the center of my collar bone, then the margins of my left and right shoulders. I bow my head, lean forward in the pew: *Lamb of God, you take away the sins of the world, have mercy on us . . .*

The church is all white stucco and wooden beams and filtered light falling from the ceiling onto the burnished pews. Above the bent body of Christ on the cross is a window painted with a white lamb and thorns, all the orange glass lit up like it's on fire as the late afternoon pours through. Logically, I know that the lamb with curled legs in the window looks like the one on Frances's gravestone only because both designs use the same available stock image for "lamb," but I can't get over how close she feels. *Lamb of God, you take away the sins of the world, have mercy on us . . .*

The priest divides the host and my gaze ricochets up and down between the crucifix and the window: *Bent body, lamb. Bent body, lamb. Bent body, lamb.*

Lamb of God, you take away the sins of the world, grant us peace . . .

*

We keep going to church, and by early fall we're staying not just for Mass, but for the weekly spaghetti dinner and the Rite of Christian Initiation for Adults sessions that are a prerequisite for conversion to the Catholic Church. Kate, a little overwhelmed by just how involved the whole process is, starts referring to RCIA as *how-to-be-Catholic class*. The directness of the phrase appeals to me, as does the sense that it might offer a blueprint for how to be faithful. How to stop the cruel and shaking fear that overtakes me sometimes, and feel closer to whatever portion of my sister outlasted her early death.

Sometimes, I feel like a tourist in church, like I lack the discipline or selflessness or certainty for real devotion and just want the trappings: the lovely church, the chorus of voices, the candlelight and the ritual and the firm hand taking mine. But I'm fond of those great lines in Andre Dubus's "A Father's Story": *Having to face and forgive my own failures, I have learned from them both the necessity and the wonder of ritual.* His protagonist muses that *a prayer, whether recited or said with concentration, is always an act of faith.*

So I say the prayers, and I go to class, and I try to take directions. I come to find St. John's church community steadying not just spiritually, but on a daily, worldly level. I'm comfortable sitting at the plastic tables in the church basement and eating big-batch spaghetti and iceberg lettuce and drinking sweet tea. I love the little girls in flowered leggings wielding washcloths heavy with the scent of industrial cleaner as they help their parents clean up. I like that they're smiling and don't look at anyone like they're a stranger. I like that our priest looks a little like Stanley Tucci, has an easy Mississippi drawl, and refers to SEC football in his homilies. The space has no pretensions and makes me want to be a more generous version of myself. *I want to be a light in the world,* I think. I feel a little less alone every week we go. And it gets easier and easier to say my prayers with devotion: make the air heat up.

But I can't enact many of the gestures the Catholic Mass requires. I can't genuflect before the altar or stand up steadily long enough to cross myself with holy water. I can't stand or kneel when the liturgy requires it, and every time I watch the congregation file up to take communion, I think about how hard that procession will be for me when I'm confirmed. I find some workarounds: I sit on the very edge of the pew and lean forward to approximate kneeling, and I work hard on my posture when the congregation is supposed to stand. I can bow quickly instead of genuflect, and Kate takes easily to crossing us both with holy water and squeezing my hand hard after she files up to get blessed by our priest, sharing with me a little of his grace.

One week, a man in the pew in front of me notices I'm not kneeling during communion and asks if I'm okay.

Yeah, I say quietly, *I just can't.*

Oh, he replies, *I thought maybe you were just too hot or something*. It's very warm in the church. I'm embarrassed.

When Mass is over, Kate leans down, grinning, and whispers in my ear, *Girl! You too* hot *to kneel*. I dissolve into hysterics and after that, it's our joke: *Girl! You too* hot *to* _____.

Really, though, I'm struggling. Is it absurd to adhere to a religion whose most central rituals my body won't let me perform? What am I to make of all the parables in the New Testament where Jesus heals the crippled and the lame? And, most importantly, if I believe we'll all eventually be resurrected back into the world, then is this body—this bruised, broken, wreck of a form—the one I'm stuck with for all time?

I've always laughed at the fanatics who occasionally come up to me on the street and offer to lay hands on me and heal my maladies. It's utterly ridiculous, and more than a little offensive, but I won't pretend that being healed isn't a dream I've had since childhood.

*

God finds ways to answer my questions. I can't believe I've become the kind of person who can write such a sentence, but there it is. One week, Father Joe gives an entire homily on the importance of Christ's bodily suffering, and the ways in which our own bodies often bear the marks of our struggles, and our sacrifices, and our striving. *What looks most like a blemish*, he says, *is often a reminder of holiness and of the Lord.*

The next week, in class, he discusses the anointing of the sick and clarifies that Christ only heals your marred body if it's necessary for the salvation of your soul. *We all have the bodies we're meant to have*, he says. *We all have the bodies we're meant to have.* What does it mean if my body is not a punishment or a mistake?

I go home and pray the rosary. *Maybe I don't have to hate my body?* I say it aloud just to test it in my mouth: *I don't have to hate my body.*

I close my eyes and picture our church: Christ's bent body on the cross, picture of a lamb.

Bent body. Lamb.

*

To prepare for my Confirmation, I go to confession the Thursday before Easter. It isn't glamorous or dark the way the movies would have you believe. It doesn't smell like sandalwood, and there are no flickering candles casting holy shadows on the walls. *I want this to be beautiful,* I think. *I feel like it would be easier if it were beautiful.* Instead, Father Joe and I sit face to face in folding chairs under florescent lights, and he smiles at me. At first, I talk in generalities, avoid what's difficult: I'm too motivated by physical beauty. I'm prone to gossip and to judgement. I like food and drink to the point of gluttony. But I work my way up to my greatest shame: I fear that my anger at God, and my body, has made me selfish and sometimes even wicked. I lay out a litany of ways I have been cruel throughout my life, ending with that July my mother and I lay in bed and I hurt her just so I could watch her hurt, just so someone else would be in pain alongside me.

I hated her, I say. *I hated God. I swore he wasn't real.*

*

When we're confirmed in the church, we pick a saint's name. I know from the first time Father Joe mentions it that I want to pick *Francis* and hear the altered echo of my sister's name inside my own.

It's not until after confession that I feel like I can say that aloud to anyone.

Bent body. Lamb.

Easter Sunday, I don't give a damn about my faltering body stumbling down the aisle toward the Eucharist.

From now on, you will be called Francis.

Bent body. Lamb.

I am fearfully and wonderfully made.

WHAT WE ARE

Lost somewhere in my parents' house in Virginia, there is an old home video of me at four- or five-years-old. I'm at a table in some occupational therapist's office, practicing drawing a circle. I hold the marker in my whole fist and move it like it's made of lead. Gently, my therapist reaches over and tries to put her hand around mine and guide it. Without a word, I shake her off. Then I reach into the basket of markers and take a new one. I look at her, give her the second pen, and move her hands forcefully toward her side of the table, shaking my head. Then I turn back to my own page, my green not-a-circle; I pick up my marker and bear down hard, concentrating. Here the camera starts to shake a little, and somewhere off-screen you can hear my father laughing.

I've been thinking a lot, lately, about the mechanisms by which we become who we are.

For instance, I was born three months early. My brain is damaged; my muscles are spastic; it has always been this way. For instance, in college I decided that I wanted to be the kind of person who drank her coffee black. So I did, cups of the stuff. I choked it down, hating it. Until, one day, I didn't anymore. This morning I drank my coffee strong and straight in the semi-dark. It wasn't a performance. For instance, my younger brother has a little extra piece of a chromosome. It doesn't have any obvious effect. It's just a fact in him that might mean something later. And, although I talk to my father several times a week, he always answers the phone, *Are you okay?*, afraid each time my siblings and I call that we're in trouble, that we've been hurt.

I always set my glass down too close to the edge of the table. I have a head for poems but not for equations, or directions, or dates. My earliest whole memory is of lying in a hospital choosing which flavor anesthetic gas I wanted to breathe while the surgeons put me under: cherry, butterscotch, grape. Or maybe it's my father reading "Those Winter Sundays"; I don't know which comes first. I still can't eat butterscotch; something in it makes me afraid.

I am an identical twin. Or was. (What's the right tense for having the same genetic material as a ghost?) My mother regularly dreams that she has forgotten one of her children somewhere in the woods. Also, she dislikes cilantro and has beautiful, illegible handwriting and no idea how the internet operates. My older sister can pick up any instrument and discern the way it works in minutes, pick out basic chord progressions like she already speaks the language. She runs marathons, pushing her body like a hot, humming engine turning over and over and over. Our little brother adores her. He can name every baseball prospect eligible for the draft this year, and when he's upset, his face sets hard just like our father's, and he doesn't want to talk to you. My father can remember no poems but all the lyrics to "Born to Run." He doesn't go to church but keeps a medal of St. Lucy hanging in his car to stand guard over his failing eyes.

Which of these things begets another? By what logic do they come into the world? How much shaping of ourselves can we do before we throw up our hands and are carried away by the sea?

*

For someone who is so clearly physically fragile, who so frequently can't get along without the help of other people, I am especially bad at being vulnerable. What I mean is, I will roll through the airport in my wheelchair with the strap of my bag in my teeth rather than let someone push me. No, what I mean is, I have a thousand-watt, *I've got it* smile. No, I'm skirting the whole truth again—what I mean is that almost every person I have ever loved has at some point looked me in the eye and said: *You have to let me in; you have to tell me what you're feeling; you have to ask for help.* Far too often I have let things go to rubble rather than open up.

*

Until the year I turn twenty-one, I somehow manage to think

my anger is a secret, a small stone only I can feel settled heavy in my throat.

That year, I'm living in Texas and teaching creative writing at an inner-city elementary school several afternoons a week. My kids are in fourth grade, but they do not know the difference between a noun, a verb, and an adjective. Many of them cannot put a sentence together. Most of them don't speak English as a first language. They associate writing with feeling dumb, and from the first day, it's clear to me that they're furious about the hours that we spend together each week. They think they've been dumped with me because they're struggling or because their parents, working long hours, are not free to pick them up when the school day ends. They're not wrong.

They refuse to pick up their pencils. They throw paper airplanes at my head. They steal each other's shoes and leap out of their seats at every available opportunity. They call me *bitch* with a casual venom that stuns me. They slap each other outright. They cry at the slightest provocation, and otherwise they yell. They are all bluster and devastation. Tiny storms. Microbursts.

There are nineteen of them. I'm a year out of college and completely lost, enraged to discover that I muscled through a childhood and adolescence marked by surgical intervention and constant physical therapy in pursuit of some bright and "better" future, only to find myself staring down the barrel of an adulthood that looks just as lonely, complicated, and medically uncertain. My knees and elbows and ankles throb. I resist the urge to yell, *Fuck you! I'm angry, too!*

But, amid the chaos, the kids are also hugely imaginative and gregarious and inventive. They stand up on chairs and share all the details of what they ate for lunch or why they hate vanilla pudding. They tell me the dreams they have about space travel robots and their ideas for the best possible superhero, who would shoot chocolate from his mouth. They want me to call them by the names of '90s pop stars I have no idea how they've ever heard of. For a week, Salvador only answers to J-Lo. Kimani ends every writing prompt we ever do with a list of all the impossibly fancy cars he wants to own: *Bugatti, Lamborghini, Ferrari, Corvette.*

One day, when I stand up briefly at the board to write an example sentence, I trip and fall down. They all rush toward me in a collective wave. Warm little bodies, tiny hands patting my back. *I fall down sometimes, too,* Jerry says matter-of-factly. Like, *Don't worry, you're not the only one.* They nod soberly.

They deserve someone so much better than me. Someone able-bodied. Experienced. Not so busy falling apart. But I'm all they've got for these small hours. I resist the urge to cry, to say, *I'm sorry. I'm sorry. I'm so sorry.*

One day, Trevor, when I tell him he has to open his notebook and get to work, looks me straight in the face and begins to stab himself in the chest with his pencil. Hard. I hear the lead break below his clavicle. He blinks tears out of his huge, brass eyes. I have never before felt quite so limited by my wheelchair. I cannot fit between the desks to reach him. I stagger up and trip in the distance between us. Inside me, something seethes. Inside me, some feral animal claws at my ribcage, trapped.

That night I go out to dinner with a friend. Talking about some article I read on the internet about how we process grief, I say: *I mean, if I had to pick a negative emotion to feel—fear, anger, sadness—I'd pick—*

Anger. You'd pick anger.

She cuts me off like she's saying: *I know. Of course you would. Of course.* She means it fondly, but there it is. I'm shocked. I ask if she thinks I am an angry person. She looks at me like I'm a lunatic.

Molly, of course. You're one of the angriest people I know.

She's kind enough to list all the other, better things she thinks I am as well. But down there with it all, she says, there's rage.

I am not keeping my own secrets especially well.

*

I learned early to love that I was fierce. To understand that my willingness to go to battle was a star under which I would thrive. You need a lot of grit, a little rage to wrestle pain. The story goes that I came into the world blue and tiny and sparring for my place in it. Two pounds, with my fists up. *Watch out,* the nurses said. *Watch out, you've got a fighter.*

What comes first: the fierceness or the need to be fierce?

Fighting, I re-learned to walk four times; I clenched my teeth through spasms. I eased dissolving stitches out of the backs of my legs. I bled inside plaster casts and muscled my body into strange cities. And I learned to spin the terror of falling down in the shower, or alone on a rainy street, into something harder-edged that would let me do much more complicated things alone. I am the woman leaping off the high dive, even when it looks like falling.

I feel an enormous amount of loyalty to the little girl in that lost home video. I see how madly she wants her own independent life, how hard she's willing to work for it, how important she already knows it is that she can make it for herself. And so I worked hard to turn her into a woman who won't back down, one who has options available to her and the gumption to go after them. One who knows how to drink whiskey and hold a political debate, wear red lipstick and fight the impulse to hate herself, however flawed and incapable she feels every day. I worked to give her everything I could of the life she wanted, miles farther from home than anybody thought she'd ever go.

Feel fear? Feel sadness? Feel lonely or wounded? If you can turn it into rage, you can use it as fuel. Get mad and you'll get up in the morning.

But somehow I've become a person who speaks sharply to everyone around her. Who wants to scream at children, then break down in tears. Whose rage is always written on her face.

You're one of the angriest people I know.

Anger is part of the engine that makes things happen, but it's savage and dangerous. It also burns things down.

I never meant to turn that girl into a forest fire.

*

Toward the end of the year, I read my class a version of Rudyard Kipling's story "How The Camel Got His Hump." I have them make construction paper signs with all the animal names and act it out on the rug in the front of the classroom, saying *humph* just like the camel does in the story, hanging their heads in frustration like the dog and the ox. They compete to see who can *humph* louder. They draw pictures of purple polka-dotted camels. I've given up on making them stay seated while we're working. Instead, I say, *One foot has to be touching your desk at all times.* They stretch their ankles as far from their bodies as possible and stick their tongues out at me. I pop a wheelie in my chair and they holler like we're at the X Games.

The next time we meet, I coax them into working on the story of how the wizard got her magic. We go sentence by sentence.

How does the wizard get her powers? *A magic asteroid!*

What is her name? *Alice the Wiz!*

Who is the enemy? *A zombie that wants to get the wizard's power by eating her brain!*

Where is it set? *A mansion!*

Write one important thing about Alice that you might not know if you looked at her? *She just wants to be happy! No, she's afraid of spiders!*

And at the end of class Julie looks up and says, *You tricked us into writing a whole story!*

Yeah! they chorus and nod their heads. They are thrilled.

Every class they ask if I'm mad at them; they ask for jelly beans. Every class they ask if I'm coming back.

*

Now, a few years later, it's early in the morning. I'm twenty-something years old in my apartment in another place I gunned hard for, and I'm trying to put my fists down. I'm weary. I'm the wildest combination of young and old. I don't want fifty more years running on rage.

The thing about the girl in that old home video? She's stubborn, and she's mad as hell, but she's smart about it. She's gentle when she shakes the therapist off. She gives the person trying to help her her own marker to use. And what's written on that girl's face when she turns back to the work of the circle on her page isn't rage, but attention.

The thing about Alice the Wiz? She just wants to be happy.

Love as fiercely as you fight. What an obnoxiously necessary platitude. Some fine thread of devotion has always run through everything I do. It's tiny and shining and down there somewhere, even overgrown by rage. It's the only reason I've ever made anything.

On my last day in the classroom with my kids in Texas, I ask them to make lists of all the things they love: *mama, Church's Chicken, Bugattis, bunny rabbits, Grand Theft Auto, my sister, being able to whistle, Captain America, the rain when it's summer.* They read them in a crazy loud chorus. I close my eyes and try to hear it.

I don't want to burn things down. But I'm suspicious of resolutions, so I'll just say this: This morning I woke up early, when Mississippi was still cold. I made my coffee and drank it black and remembered that I had made that possible for myself. I watched the sun come up and loved the light and concentrated on feeling happy.

Hey, stubborn little blond-haired girl, we won. We are alive. And now the work is to be gentler with ourselves and with the world. I want such a sweet life for you. I want the fierceness of attention, of the light coming over the hill, of your own hand bringing a cup to your mouth. Of love, which will abide so much longer than the fire.

NARRATIVE AND NEED

About a year ago, I published a collection of poems that got a little attention. Not the kind that turns authors into celebrities or lands a book on any bestseller lists, not even enough to make a novelist turn her head, but a dizzying amount for a young poet. People who weren't obligated by either blood or friendship actually bought copies; the book got a couple of major reviews; I did some radio interviews and, all of a sudden, I had invitations to read at colleges and conferences all over the country. I've spent large swaths of the last year in row twenty-two of some little airplane watching the perfect grids of cities come into focus below me: Nashville, Baltimore, Houston, Chicago, Grand Forks, St. Louis. I unpack and repack my bag on the impossibly white sheets of some Marriott, Hilton, Homewood Suites. I read in a library; give a talk in a corner classroom; marvel every time at the nickel-bright faces of the students in front of me, the urgency of their questions, the fact of them all there, holding my book in their hands. I go out to dinner with graduate students or faculty, ask about their projects, stay quiet a long time listening to the answers. When I should, I tell a joke; the table laughs. I'm good in public. I board another plane.

This is the thing I've always wanted: to write something that weighs enough to leave a mark wherever it's set down, to get to watch it working out there in the world. When people ask, I say that I feel lucky and also tired. That I wake up in the mornings and sometimes, for a second, can't remember where I am. That all of it feels like this impossible gift: these places, everyone I'm meeting, and these regular reminders that, somehow, there are people out there touched by the thing I've made. And it's true, I'm *grateful,* and exhausted, and so happy that I'm sure everyone can hear joy humming underneath my skin.

What I don't say to anyone is that, also, late at night, when I'm the only passenger on a little white bus tearing through the back roads of New Jersey like they're water, I feel a flash of worry that this is really the only kind of life I'm suited for: set down someplace just long enough to make a good impression, gone before the shine of me wears off. Best known only briefly, as a city in outline, blinking in the far-off distance.

*

A need is a requirement, a necessity. But once upon a time, need also meant, *violence, force, constraint, or compulsion exhibited by or on someone.* Need like a hammer. Need like a rope around the neck.

*

When my father calls to tell me his mother has died, my book is still a pile of manuscript pages on an editor's desk. I'm in a graduate seminar and don't pick up the phone, although I see the screen light up on the table beside me. I know why he's calling. She's been in the hospital for days. I wait to call him back until I'm headed home from campus. It's evening, and the February light is going and blue. I press the phone tightly to my ear.

My father is known for volume. In his classroom, he shouts at his students, and they love him for it. Making a point, he slams his hand down on the table in enthusiasm. He sneezes and the lightbulb shudders in the overhead lamp. He turns the stereo all the way up; he can't *believe* you've never heard this song. But when he's sad, or has to tell you something difficult, his voice is pitched so quiet that it's often hard to hear it. Someone told me once that, when you listen to a whisper, your eardrum moves a fraction of the width of an atom. It's one of those stupidly beautiful pieces of trivia that's almost certainly wrong, and I think about it every time I hear my father's voice go soft: this fragile, essential thing, shifting invisibly.

When we talk, he tells me that my siblings know already, and then says, *I knew this would be hardest for you.* He means that, in the story of our family, I'm the one who every feeling comes the hardest for—who, as a child, howled for three days straight when my parents sold our beat-up Honda, who buried every small, dead, wild thing the woods turned up, who was moved first to tears, and tenderness, and rage. But he means, too, that I keep my grandfather's rosary looped on my dresser, that I'm the one who keeps in some small touch with both his sisters, that one July he and I drove alone from Virginia to New Orleans, and for a week I asked him just to take me through the city as he'd known it: the neighborhood where he was raised—still partly empty nearly a decade after Hurricane Katrina; his Jesuit school; the Crippled Children's Hospital where his father worked; the bar where he'd get high school drunk on bad Tequila Sunrises; the family mausoleum. I'm the one who takes notes. Who worries over the record. Over his silences. I met his mother maybe five or six times in my life. When I ask him how he's feeling, now, he pauses, says, *I think, mostly relieved. She isn't suffering anymore. She can't make anyone else suffer.*

*

The first time I see a psychiatrist alone I'm maybe seven, and I've stopped sleeping through the night. I fall asleep fine, but I wake up screaming in the dark, gripped by fear that something terrible has happened to everyone I love; that someone has come in through the unlocked door of my family's farmhouse and killed my mother and my father and both my sleeping siblings and that right now he is creeping toward my room to come and pin me down and shoot me, too. During the day I'm angry and sullen. I don't want to do the exercises the physical therapist has assigned to help keep me mobile. I don't want to do anything. My parents are worried, and devoted, and would like to be able to sleep through the night themselves. *Just talk to him,* they urge me. I see that psychiatrist on and off until I go to junior high. I make fake meals in a plastic kitchen. I beat on a tiny red punching bag. I arrange army men in swift, haphazard groups and knock them down with the heel of my hand. I talk the whole length of every appointment: I'm angry at my body, which hurts, at my legs, which buckle and won't hold me when I want them to. I don't want to have cerebral palsy. I don't want my parents to have to hold me up or help me climb into the bath. I don't want to need them even in the ways the therapist assures me all children need their parents. I want them to disappear. I'm still dreaming that they disappear. I don't want to need anything, from anyone, ever.

On the elementary school playground, I'm unable to keep up with my classmates playing four square or tag or scaling the old fireman's pole. I'm tired of sitting alone on a bench. And so, instead, I sit down at the edge of the woods on the playground's scrubby outlying corner. I mark a boundary with nearby sticks, and I tell my classmates that, if they want, they can come tell me their problems. I tell them soberly that it's my job to listen. And, for weeks, they really do come. Enough of them to form a small, unwieldy line at the sticks I've laid down. They come to talk about their younger siblings, the pets they want, the fights they have with their best friend, their frustrations with their parents. I don't remember the details of what any of them said or what I said to them in return. I think that it was very little, that mostly I listened. I do remember that they often said thank you. That I felt important and powerful, like I'd hit on a trick. I could make myself necessary. They were *waiting* to talk to me. I was very, very glad not to be alone.

My parents are both novelists, and my family of storytellers loves this story. *Just the same person she's always been. So resourceful. So curious. Such a good listener.* I like this story in the same way, if I don't think too hard about it. If I spend too much time reflecting I think: *Just the same person I've always been,* and hate myself a little.

*

My family is a close one, and we make our lives in language. Even my siblings, who aren't writers by trade, have the storytelling gene. They work in politics and business: charming and articulate, schooled in knowing how to convey exactly what they mean. Being raised in the house of novelists manifests itself in all ways you might expect: My parents read to us for years, long past the age where we could read on our own. There are books on every available surface, and beyond them. Family lore is particularly polished, and my parents prized our childhood dinner conversation, often asked: *Tell us about your day in detail?* Or, *Describe that more?* My father played a game with us where he would offer up a word and ask us for the opposite, making each set progressively more nuanced: What *is* the exact opposite of *anguished*? Not quite *happy* or *relieved*. It wasn't until I applied to graduate school that I realized this is an exercise lifted right out of the verbal section of the GRE.

But the primacy of language in our lives manifests in ways that are subtler than that, too. My family almost never hangs up the phone, or leaves the house, without saying *I love you*. Something important in the constant articulation, even when it's mostly reflex. This sense that something grows realer when you put it in language. Only as an adult did I discover that my siblings, too, keep almost every card or letter they've ever received, no matter how inconsequential, no matter how impractical the practice. Like there's something almost sacrilegious in throwing away what, even for a second, mattered enough to someone to write down.

My family talks about almost everything, and so the few things consigned mostly to silence loom particularly large in the absence of a shared language for them: Twenty-seven years after her death, I've never heard my father say my twin sister's name. My mother and I talk about her only rarely. Their grief at her loss is too difficult and feral to shape a story from. My father's childhood, too, I infer largely from the shape his silence takes around it.

My father is the fifth of eight children born in ten years. Six boys and then two girls raised not too far from Lake Pontchartrain in New Orleans. His father had a paralyzed leg from a bike accident as a boy and was a local orthopedic surgeon, busy and beloved by his patients. Kind, but mostly absent. He died when I was four. I don't remember him, although my father says he called more after I was born, that we spoke on the phone even when I was too young to really converse. He was fond of some linkage, maybe, in our damaged bodies. It's one of the few details about his family that my father likes to recount.

His mother was distant, perennially angry, and ugly-cold to the point of cruelty, though I don't know if she hit her children with any regularity. My father doesn't volunteer specifics and, in rare moments when I try to press him, just goes soft, then silent. But I know he knew how to make her a gin and tonic before he turned ten, and that he never thought she loved him. We saw her occasionally when I was very young, and then almost never after my grandfather died. She sent generic cards at holidays, and occasionally sent my parents money when they were desperate, although it always made something look ruined in my father if he had to ask. He'd be stormy and unreachable for days.

My father couldn't ever bear for us to be angry with him. My mother did almost all the disciplining when we were growing up, and the only time my father got involved was when we treated our mother badly. *You have no idea how lucky you are*, he'd hiss, the kind of angry that made everything about him shake. And then his voice, that particular quiet, *no idea how lucky.*

*

I go to college at sixteen and, over the next few years, become an expert at falling in with people who fall apart in spectacularly dramatic ways. There are worrying numbers of pills and the seizures they bring on. There are ambulance rides, long silent spells, and weeping fights. I spend hours in the emergency room late at night during finals week, and I neglect my own homework and necessary trips to the gym because instead I'm comforting a boy who won't get out of bed, or holding a girl's hair back out of her face when she vomits. I am watching a friend all the time, like the ER doctor told us to, until she can get an appointment to see a neurologist. I am crying in my own room with my knees pressed to my chest.

My life is also full of steadier friends, people who cook dinner and ask questions, care for me and make me laugh.

My parents and family are constant and loving. But I share very little about my own inner life with anyone, and as little about my body as I can get away with. *I don't want to need anything, from anyone, ever.*

It's not until I'm twenty-one and back in therapy, trying to pick up the pieces after having been forced to leave my first attempt at graduate school, lied about it to everyone for months, and terrified the people who love me by finally self-destructing in my own awful fashion, that I take seriously the suggestion that these two things are probably related. That my pathological fear of needing anyone for anything at all—of failing in any way, real or imagined—is linked to my insatiable desire to make myself indispensable, to find people I can get busy saving. That all of this stems from a belief that I can't trust anyone's affection if it isn't born of need.

*

I meet my parents in New Orleans for my grandmother's funeral. It's a quick flight from Mississippi, and the night before the service my father and I drink complicated, expensive cocktails in the hotel bar and mostly don't talk. He has very little to say that weekend, although he thanks my mother and me again and again for being there with him, as if we would be anywhere else.

The next morning, we have hours in the church before the funeral Mass starts, and I mill around making small talk and trying to look busy. My father and his seven siblings are each there with a partial collection of their children, and I keep thinking how remarkable it is that I'm related to this many people I hardly know at all. I'm not sure I could name all of my cousins if I tried. My father and his siblings all seem to have remarkably good family lives given how much damage their mother did, but their steadiness seems largely predicated on not having a substantive relationship with one another or acknowledging certain facts of their childhood. And my father, something in him particularly fragile and damaged, holds himself at an especially far remove.

I only really remember spending time with my grandmother once: the summer I turned twenty-two and my father and I made that drive alone to New Orleans. We stopped on the way at the retirement community in Birmingham where she'd moved after the hurricane and took her to dinner. She was barely walking by then, shuffling around with a walker, looking pained. My father asked, *Mama,* the word sounding unnatural when he spoke it, *have you ever thought about getting a wheelchair? It might make things easier for you.* She looked right at me, then, sitting in my own wheelchair in the doorway of her apartment, and said, *Oh, I could never, it would be too sad.* And I didn't know her well enough to know whether to read cruelty or pity in her voice, or to believe that, somehow, she really wasn't thinking about me at all. We took a photograph together on her couch, and later, while my father loaded the car, the old landline in her living room rang, and she asked me to pick it up. The voice on the line asked if I was Mrs. Brown, and I said, *No, this is Mrs. Brown's granddaughter,* a phrase I've only used that once. When I asked who was inquiring, it was only the Republican Party, calling as part of a fundraiser. I never saw her again.

The funeral Mass, once it starts, is long and strained. My mother calls the priests presiding the *lost boys,* and they do look somehow stray and stranded up there in their collars. I learn a handful of things about my grandmother that I didn't know: that her middle name was Joy, that she ran a reading group for Catholic women in New Orleans and captained regular charity drives and working groups; that she gave a not-small sum of money to advocate for permitting women to be Catholic priests. No one who talks about her calls her kind or gentle. They call her *organized, smart.* Half the people who speak use only platitudes, the others say she could be, well, *intimidating.* It's clear to me that she was a stranger to everyone here, including her children, and that she's left them relative strangers to one another, and I can't decide if I feel sad or angry in greater measure. The whole thing makes me want to cry, or scream, but I don't want my father to feel like he needs to comfort me. I bite the inside of my cheek instead.

It's only when we're at the cemetery that we learn my grandmother has asked not to be buried in the family mausoleum, with her husband and the generations before them. Instead, she wants to be cremated and placed in a slot of the wall at the far side of the cemetery, near the huge plot of some local fried chicken mogul and no one she knows. She'd like, she said, *some peace and quiet.*

I knew it, my father will say to my mother and me later, shaking his head quickly back and forth. *I knew her whole life all she wanted was for us to leave her alone. I was right,* he says, and then again like he can't believe he has proof now, *I was right.*

When the day is mostly over, and it's just my mother and me for a few minutes, I do lose my composure and start crying. The silent, torrential kind of tears. *Molly, what is it?* My mother says, bewildered, *I don't understand why you're this upset.* And I don't know how to explain how heartbroken I feel that my father is mostly relieved his mother is dead, and how much I hate knowing that all that potential for anger and estrangement is *in* me somehow. That it runs in my blood. That I'm part of it.

*

The truth is that my grandmother was twenty-five, married, and middle-class Catholic in the early 1950s, continuously pregnant for the better part of a decade, then expected to stay home and raise her children. Granted another kind of life in another moment, she might have chosen to have one child, or none. To be a social worker or a professor, an activist or female priest. She might have been happier, might have been kinder, might have been known. I wish her that freedom. But she felt backed into a corner by her circumstances, by the story of her life, and so she was cold-hearted and vicious, dying a stranger to the people who should have known her best because she couldn't make her peace with what there was no changing, because she couldn't trust anyone enough to let them love her.

*

My father asks me to promise that I'll have nicer things to say about him at his funeral—that he's done a good job loving me. My gentle, loud, funny, fragile, impossibly devoted father, who looks old to me in the low light of the restaurant. Whose eyes are failing. And I say, *Yes. Of course. I love you. And you're not allowed to die anytime soon.*

I want to ask him to promise the same thing back. But that's an absurd request, so I just take his hand across the table.

*

Now, in my present life, my apartment in Arkansas is only mine for a few more weeks. I don't own any of the furniture. I moved in less than a year ago, and I've spent so much time on book tour that I've rarely been here longer than a few weeks at a time. Soon, I'll get on another plane, and in a couple of months, I'm leaving for a year in a city where I don't speak the language. I'm almost twenty-seven, and I have no children, no husband—and no promise of either on the horizon. My life is the opposite of my grandmother's life. I want every piece of this adventure. It scares me how often everyone around me is a stranger.

Sometimes at night, in a new hotel, I put myself to sleep by listing all the people whom I really love; all the people who I know and trust know me; the little list I'm working on of people I allow myself to need.

The Skin You're In

In Italian, the verb "to skin" is *spellare*. The way I understand it, this is a verb distinct from the Italian for *peel*, or *strip*, or *shuck*. It's the word you'd use for preparing an animal, for flaying a corpse. Informally, you can also use a version of it when you mean *I skinned my knee* or even *I shed my skin*. Either way, it's a word that connotes a body revealed and ready for refashioning. I learn all this one afternoon in Bologna at the threshold of the Anatomical Theater of the Archiginnasio, a friend translating the librarian's rapid Italian as quickly as she can manage. We're at the first site of the University of Bologna's medical school, and this room—built in 1637— is where they taught the earliest human anatomy courses and did some of the first sanctioned dissections of human bodies in the West. Surgery, as we understand it, was essentially born here, and now the librarian is gesturing up at the wall above the marble operating table, where two lacquered wooden statues gaze down. I look closer and realize they're all carved visible muscle and bone. He calls them *Spellati: the skinless ones.*

This trip is a colossal, improbable gift. My first collection of poems has just been released and, as part of its publication, I'm here in Italy to spend six weeks at an artist's residency at a castle in Umbria. I'm twenty-five and about three weeks out of graduate school. The notion that I have any kind of a writing career still feels a little like a joke, and when you combine it with words like *castle* and *Europe* and *funded fellowship*, I have the distinct sensation I am watching a movie of someone else's life. I can't stop fingering the passport in my purse; I need a constant, tangible reminder that this is really happening. I can't believe my own luck.

But, over the last year or so, as my book has come into being and my professional life has come to resemble more and more the one I've been dreaming of since I was a child, my body has been undergoing its own kind of transformation. The symptoms of my cerebral palsy are worsening. Recently, the low consistent ache in my knees has been increasing in intensity and my back has begun to spasm whenever I stand up. Hard enough to knock me over if I'm not careful. The two kinds of changes form a mystifying syncopated rhythm: I have a piece of artistic good luck and, as if in concert, I get a little less mobile, am in a little more pain. I use my wheelchair more and more, even for very short distances.

In the two weeks before I leave for Italy, I push myself too hard while preparing to travel. I take a nasty fall and wrench something I can feel but not name. All of a sudden it hurts when I'm sitting at my desk, when I roll over in bed, when I bend to tie my shoes. I'm panicked and enraged at the timing. I drag myself to the doctor and ask for a cortisone shot and a prescription for a heavy-duty muscle relaxer I can take on the ten-hour plane ride to Italy. The doctor at the campus health center wants to request my medical records, wants to do an x-ray and figure out what's really going on. *I don't have time,* I tell him, *I have things to do.* He shakes his head but gives me the shot and the prescription.

I want to tell him, *Listen, I'm breaking every rule I've ever had for how I treat my body.* I'm suspicious of quick fixes, steroids, narcotics, anything that masks the real weather of the body with false calm. I want to say, *I swear I've been tender; I've been tough when I needed to be; I've let my body call the shots so it would last. Just this once, I need to force it to fall in line.* I want to make him understand: *I love my body, but I can't let it take this from me.*

Instead, I say *thank you,* and leave his office gingerly.

*

Here, in Bologna, I'm visiting an old friend for a few days before my residency starts, and we've come into the anatomical theater through a circuitous back entrance in a connected building, one that involves an elevator so narrow I can barely fit my wheelchair inside it, as well as several locked doors, which the librarian leads us through apologetically. My friend translates his steady stream of apologies and explanations: *This is a very old, historic building; they had to get so many special permits even to put an elevator in the one next door; this city is terrible for people in wheelchairs; if he had known I didn't walk . . .* I've discovered, by now, that I can get almost nowhere in this city through the front door, and that there are many places I can't access at all. I've also fallen in love with the light and the occasional hidden channels of water tucked behind wrought iron gates, all the rose-colored stone, and the throng of the main piazza. The past feels shoulder to shoulder with the present here. I want to witness everything, and I'm having trouble knowing what to do with the way the magic of the place is tangled up in my inability to access it. Or with how my sense of my unbelievable luck is butting heads with my mounting anxiety about my mobility, my mounting frustration about my pain. The dissonance makes me fragile and defensive:

My life is extraordinary. How dare I feel sadder than I do grateful?

There's so much in the world I want to see and do, and already so much of it is unreachable to me.

The last time I had a sudden, inexplicable increase in pain, it marked the first time I needed a wheelchair, the last time I walked more than a city block. I never got that early body back.

This is the beginning of the life I've always wanted.
What if I'm about to lose another body?

*

Next to the spellati there are carved statues of famous physicians (Hippocrates, Galenus) flanked by renderings of Apollo, several Catholic saints, and constellations named for figures from mythology. Humanity, science, and all of these conceptions of divinity conjured up together for some sort of communion in the service of understanding how it is we're made, and what to do with that.

My own body feels skinless, rubbed raw. I imagine it, butterflied, on the marble table: brain and heart, liver and lungs, muscles and tendons all laid bare, all my brain's bad wiring in evidence, thickets of scar tissue every place a surgeon has reshaped me over the years.

*

Does it matter if I tell you that the anatomical theater itself is essentially a reconstruction? The original chamber was mostly destroyed in an air raid during the Second World War. After the bombs, they pulled the old statues from the rubble and rebuilt the place from the ground up. They tried to use as much of the original material as possible, to make it match, as closely as they could, a sturdier version of the very place that it had been before. You can't see the seams where they affixed the spellati and the saints to the new walls.

Does it matter that dissection was once considered too invasive and violent a study to subject most bodies to? That, originally, they used the corpses of criminals and prostitutes as instructive cadavers, and then buried them in unmarked graves without bothering to stitch them back together again? That, while doctors gave instructions to medical students, they left the actual cutting to butchers?

I owe the current shape of my body, almost every inch of mobility I've ever had, to scores of people taken apart without their consent, people no one cared enough to name or suture into any kind of remade whole once they had taken what they could.

The book that won me this fellowship to Italy is about a real government-run residential hospital for people with serious mental and physical disabilities that was the epicenter of the American eugenics movement in the first half of the twentieth century. More than 8,000 people were sterilized there without their knowledge. One colossal misunderstanding about the brain and the body piled on top of another; doctors with just enough knowledge about how we're made to do cataclysmic, permanent violence, spurred by terror. *Cut a body just like that to ensure that it will never make another one. Stitch like that to sew it back together.*

Does it matter that the midday light in this operating theater washes the whole place the color of dark, sweet cherries?

That, on top of their sinewy bodies, the skinless men have the fine-boned faces of angels?

How about this? In a handful of months, my health insurance will lapse. And at home, in the United States, the government is doing its level best to make me uninsurable. I have needed fixing from the moment I was born. I can feel myself falling apart. Does it matter that I am afraid?

*

In Bologna, I take the muscle relaxer every night, a heavy-duty anti-inflammatory every morning. I do everything I can to keep my body quiet, tell it, *Hush; please behave; we're so lucky to be here.* One day, I climb five tall flights of stairs, leaning heavily on a railing, because I have to reach the top of a nearby city. Everybody says it's an unmissable view, so I have to see it now in case I never can again. In case it's my last chance to ever climb this high. It's extraordinary, all those terracotta roofs spilling beautifully down the green mountain. The walls of fortresses and spires of churches punctuating an otherwise empty sky.

I can't do it justice; you'd have to see it for yourself.

That night, I don't really sleep. My hips and knees ache so intensely I can almost hear it. I lie still on the mattress because any real motion produces a spasm. Maybe you can only ask your body to lie to itself for so long.

And so, once I get to Umbria and my residency begins

in earnest, I taper off the medication, don't get up out of the wheelchair except to walk a couple of steps to the dinner table, or climb gingerly into a golf cart, or a car. *Okay*, I tell my body, *you can get loud again. I'll listen. I'll be gentle.* There's so much I can't see of the castle's beautiful grounds, so many places I can't go at all. Not even once in my life.

But, out the window of my bedroom here, some foreign flower is blooming a gorgeous yellow in the courtyard below, and in the morning there are piles and piles of apricots, bright and sweet in a white china bowl. There's a tiny, retrofitted elevator in the center of the castle, and the door of the turret is *just* wide enough that I can ease my wheelchair through to see the sun set, a huge red fist above the horizon. As long as I'm gentle, the pain mostly eases to a constant tenderness. I can't believe my own luck.

I don't know exactly what's happening in my body, and I fear soon someone will need to take it apart again and stitch it back together. So I'm trying to listen as I shift inside myself, and watch the world from every angle I can see without standing. Preparing, quietly, to transform again.

You can use the verb *spellare* when you mean: *I shed my skin.*

SOMETHING'S WRONG WITH ME

The earliest lexicon I remember having available to define myself is a medical glossary of defect and attempted repair: *ruptured amniotic sac, neurological disorder, increased spasticity, impaired fine-motor control, dorsal rhizotomy, cartilage disintegration, orthopedic surgeon, orthotics, plaster molding, gait monitoring and maintenance, physical therapy, magnetic resonance imaging, double upright KFOs*. Find all cross-listed under deformity; deficiency; disability.

By kindergarten, I could tell you, in the Donald Duck voice I spoke with because I couldn't really clear my throat: *I have cerebral palsy, which is a little like a stroke that happens when you're born*. There is probably not a single other sentence I have uttered more frequently in all my years of being alive. It appears in every facet of my life, addressed at one time or another to nearly every stranger and acquaintance and friend. To the potential employer: *I have cerebral palsy, which is a little like a stroke that happens when you're born*. To the handsome, confused guy across the table in the coffee shop: *I have cerebral palsy, which is a little like . . .* To the college girl in the grocery store aisle who looks shiftily at the adapted Segway that I sometimes use to get around, the man behind me in line at the ATM who asks why I'm in a wheelchair, the mother and her little boy, the older woman coming out of church who sees my cane and my weird walk and says, *You're too beautiful to be disabled, what happened to you!?*

I have cerebral palsy . . .

One day I report an interaction like this, and a friend's surprise at a stranger's forwardness, to my father on the phone. I say: *I had to tell her this happens to me all the time.* He corrects me, out of what impulse I'm not completely sure: *Well, not all the time, but sometimes . . .* I don't remember if I force the issue, but it's true—all the time. At least once almost every time I leave my house. This is not an exaggeration.

*

There is a strange kind of security about having something so immutable at the center of yourself. Once, I was interviewed briefly for a local news segment about new adaptive technology. The caption underneath me while I spoke read: *Molly Brown: physically disabled.* It's hard to argue with this. Whatever ontological unease I feel, however ethereal my thoughts become, the truth of my body is literal and absolute, like an anchor pulling me back to the world.

And that other essential, persistent refrain is as important as ever, however often I repeat it. I am lucky—lucky to be

alive, to be as mobile and unscarred as I am, to be as independent as I am capable of being. I am lucky to have been born
to smart, devoted parents, to have received an extraordinary
education, to be able to articulate my life and my body. I am
lucky that it is possible for me to stand up, both literally and
figuratively, for myself and others like me when it's called
for. I am lucky for a million other reasons that I am not
listing here.

*

But can I admit something unflattering and exhausted and
ungenerous?

I'm so tired of talking about disability. I'm tired of talking
about its place in culture and politics. I'm tired of talking
about my body and other people's bodies, and of feeling like
leaving my house in the morning is a political act. I'm tired of,
whatever I write and whatever I'm thinking, feeling disability
bang around at the back of my brain and insist on a presence
in everything. Get out. Leave me alone. Get out. Get out.

I spent nearly the entire day yesterday sitting in front
of this computer trying not to write this essay—which I feel
like I've written a thousand versions of before—negotiating
out loud with the thick, warm air: I will write about anything
else, anything at all. There's a whole world out there, and I
spent my week imagining women slowly losing their minds
trapped in a hospital. Couldn't there be something else in my

writing mind? Last week, when a woman in the Thai restaurant where I was picking up takeout looked at my Segway and, not knowing any better, asked me if I wouldn't rather just walk, I almost said, *You bitch!* just so I wouldn't have to say, *Actually, I have cerebral palsy ...*

I'm tired of feeling left out of every conversation about femininity, and every conversation about feminism, like I can't ever find another voice in the chorus like mine, an experience that matches my own. Trying to explain this to a good friend who's recently started blogging for a feminist website, I say: nobody anywhere in the media looked anything like me when I was growing up. Nobody on television, or on any magazine cover, or in any book. Even in counterculture I couldn't find a model.

I'm not alone in feeling the impact of that silence, that lack. Introducing a recent report on disability representation in the media, Ford Foundation senior fellow Judith E. Heumann writes:

> *Growing up, I rarely, if ever, saw anyone with a disability on television or in movies. If disabled people were shown at all, they were portrayed as villains to be reviled ... or as objects of pity for charitable causes such as the Jerry Lewis Telethon and on numerous soap operas where "good" or beloved characters were apt*

to be miraculously cured of their disability. Without question, there was nobody I could look to and say, "There's a positive, high-achieving disabled person like me," and certainly no one I could look to as a role model who reflected my actual lived experience.

According to the Centers for Disease Control and Prevention, one out of every four Americans has a disability, but Heumann notes in her report that only 2.1 percent of primetime broadcast TV series regulars—a total of sixteen characters—have disabilities. In the one hundred top grossing movies of the last ten years, only 2.5 percent of characters are depicted with disabilities. Those numbers grow even more dismal and damaging if you're a disabled woman, or person of color, looking to see yourself reflected in the media around you.

The consequences of this lack of representation aren't merely intellectual or theoretical. As I aged out of childhood, nothing in my world made any room for me, warned me, or prepared me, for the life I'd have to lead. Nothing offered any advice: Here's how your disability can co-exist with your gender, your sexuality, your politics, your ambition. Here's how to talk about it to bosses and lovers, here's how not to let it get so big it drowns out everything else about you. I had to make it all up as I went along.

The ugliest, most selfish part of me is tired of feeling

responsible for the chasm I feel—like somehow I have to end it, change it, fill it up.

*

The other night, I put on a nice dress and went to a bar I don't usually frequent, but that I knew was accessible. I parked my Segway against the back wall and chose a table close enough that I could see it, but far enough away that it wasn't obviously mine. I sat in the semi-dark and drank a bourbon and enjoyed the thought that, looking at me, nobody would know, that sitting at the table right now I could be any pretty young woman with a book in a bar. For all they knew, I could go dance. I could get up and walk right out of there, painless and fluid and unremarkable. I wouldn't need to field a single comment or question, or get a single sorry look.

This lasted a few minutes, and then I felt guilty as hell for trying to crawl out of my own skin.

Later, I put off sending the email in which I have to write and tell the woman interviewing me for a job on Tuesday that I'm in a wheelchair. I worry about the mother who emailed me about tutoring her daughter in SAT prep, and then just stopped writing after I revealed I use one. Who knows what happened, but...

*

I've been seeing someone very casually for a little while, and while he's made it clear he's interested, it's also clear that he's more than a little uncomfortable with his relationship to my body: He looks down at the floor when I walk around my apartment, is reluctant to go out together in public. When we're lying on my bed and his hand finds the small snarl of scar tissue on my lower back, he flinches, pulls away. He doesn't touch me anywhere near there again.

One night, before he comes over, I catch myself wondering whether I ought to put cover-up on the bruises that dot my legs and feet from the fall I took the previous night, and trying to imagine how I can stand up as little as possible once he arrives: *If I've already poured our drinks, then . . .* It's more than wanting to be pretty, then putting on mascara or a dress that makes me look skinnier. In all of this, I'm trying to play-act not just a different body, but a different life in which this history of damage isn't mine and, on a night when he's more uncomfortable than usual, I don't need to worry that I might fall down the concrete stairs ahead of him because my pride won't let me take his arm.

And here, again, my privilege rises to the surface: My daily life is manageable enough that I have time to meditate on the cultural position of disability. When I need a night off from my body I can go to a bar and sidle away from myself, pretend to be a different kind of woman with a different existence. I can blend in, pass. And, however complicated it has been—will be—there have been people who've loved me, found me beautiful, become comfortable beside me. When I really remember all this, it is enough to begin to soothe the tired, freaked out, fucked-up part of me that's been screaming for a break.

*

The truth is, mostly, I don't want a different life or even a different body. I've brokered peace with my hair, my spade-like nails, my ghostly pale skin. My neck is my mother's neck, my face is my father's face. And this body, as complicated as it is, gave me rapt attention. It gave me empathy and maturity. It gave me discipline and poetry, and enough hurt and strangeness to really need it. And I wouldn't trade away anything that might take with it the way I fill up when I read Emily Dickinson. *After great pain, a formal feeling comes . . .*

The truth is I want the same thing so many activists work for. I want a different, better world than the one I came of age in. Each child with a disability will always know too early the dictionary of defects and treatments essential to her life. But I want for them all to have, too, another language with which to talk about their bodies and their lives: one of pride and complexity, intimacy and particularity, survival and triumph. I want them all to know that there are other bodies that look and move like theirs, bodies that aren't lying in hospital beds or aging bitterly in the corners of rooms, and I want them to have easy access to voices that will comfort and console and instruct them and welcome their presence in the chorus. I don't want them to go it alone. I want them to believe in the possibility of love, and adventure, and beauty, and a whole complete life, however trite that all sounds. And there are people out there working to make this possible, people who know the only corrective to absence, stereotyping, and silence comes when we raise our voices.

To help realize the world I want, I have to write, I have to talk. Language is my medium. It is the thing that has borne me up and out of every valley, the thing that has tied me to other people and made my life large. Often, it's the only thing I really believe in.

*

So I stop fighting with the air and write this essay. I tell the woman who's interviewing me next week what to expect. I gather myself and put my hands in my hair, lean close to that guy I'm seeing and say: *Listen, you can tell me if you're feeling uncomfortable and we'll talk about it, you can ask questions if you have them, you can take your time getting to know me, but you can't push me away like that because you're freaking out about the wheelchair. I'm done with the part of my life where I feel ashamed of myself and of my body. I'm not about to go back there, okay? That's the deal.*

And, when I'm ready, I stand up from the table in that bar. I stumble a little and stomp over to the wall. Outside, some guy at one of the tables stops me. *Hey, what's the deal with the Segway?* In a lot of ways, I'm better at this than anything else, meant for this sentence and the conversation it starts: *Hi, I use it instead of a wheelchair; I have cerebral palsy, which is . . .*

The Virginia State Colony for Epileptics and Feebleminded

Growing up in the middle of nowhere means you spend a lot of time in the car: ten miles to school or the grocery store, thirty-five to the movie theater or a decent restaurant, nearly sixty to the nearest place you might want to buy clothes. You drive the same stretch of rural highway so many thousands of times you stop seeing it, mile markers and exit signs, the constant purple rise of the Blue Ridge in the distance yawning in and out of fog. For years, I sped past Colony Road and the government-issued sign for The Central Virginia Training Center without much interest. I knew vaguely that it was a residential facility for people with serious disabilities, and that it had a complicated history, tangled up with Appalachia, eugenics, and the Great Depression. In high school, grappling with my own cerebral palsy, I sometimes thought about it glancingly, the way you consider something that *almost* relates to you but doesn't, a distant relative you've only heard stories about. Mostly, though, the facility was just another feature of the place I was raised: red clay hills, Baptist church, bakery, Training Center—all of it as unexceptional as my own hand.

I was eighteen the summer that changed, home in Virginia between my sophomore and junior years of college, taking a theology class at the university about an hour north of my hometown. Initially, I devised a day trip out to the boondocks of my childhood as a diversion for a close friend who was having a hard time. We bought cheeseburgers at McDonald's, put her dog in the truck, and turned the radio up. The plan was to go south and do a drive-by tour of my one-stoplight town, and then continue on into Bedford where we'd heard there was an attraction called *Holyland USA,* a kind of home-made theme park featuring all the stations of the cross. The trip was supposed to be easy and amusing, a chance to share the idiosyncrasies of a landscape I loved.

I don't remember, now, why we decided to turn off the highway at Colony Road. Because we'd never been there? Because the honeysuckle was blooming over the gate and looked beautiful? Because the dog was whining in the cab and needed to be let out? After the wrought-iron gate, the road forked in two directions. One led to the facility, the other to its sprawling cemetery. Like many things in central Virginia, the Training Center sits on a huge amount of land, the acreage around it much greater than you could practically ever use. As the facility fell into disrepair in the many years after its founding in the early 1900s, instead of being rehabbed or knocked down, older buildings were simply abandoned, new construction rising around them on all the available land. That day we first visited the place, it struck me as the eeriest combination of ghost town and functioning operation: at once the establishment that it is now and the shadow of everything that it had been—built up around its own troubling history in the most literal of senses.

The Training Center today makes little explicit concession to that dark past, when it was called the Virginia State Colony for Epileptics and Feebleminded. There's a small sign out front that acknowledges the old name. And on the facility's website, a page marked *history* includes, just after a discussion of the Colony's first post office, a single paragraph explaining that for a period, in accordance with Virginia law, "the facility embarked on an ill-advised program of involuntary sterilization, combined with routine appendectomies, of so-called '... defectives with cacogenic potentialities.'" That's all there is. No details about the men and women who once filled the infirmary beds, or the salpingectomies and vasectomies performed without their consent or even their knowledge.

That July day, we drove slowly through the Training Center's grounds, my wheelchair rattling like animal bones in the truck bed. The buildings were a mix of brick and white clapboard, the older ones slouching like ragged, hollow ghosts next to the center's contemporary facilities, marked with black numbers that no longer seemed to indicate any kind of order. We didn't talk much, but I hung half my body out the passenger side window, looking at the white-washed porches and the cloudy windows—in which sometimes a stray curtain still hung—and counting the *crossing for handicapped pedestrians* signs. Occasionally, we saw a maintenance truck, but whoever lived there seemed shut away inside. No one stopped us to ask who we were.

Eventually, we parked down by the cemetery and got out. I pulled my wheelchair from the truck but quickly abandoned it. The wheels stuck in the gravel and the clay. I leaned on my friend's arm, or put my palms to the dirt where the hills were high to keep my balance. We picked our way toward the outlying buildings and the flat grave-markers lain into the hill. The stones were dated as early as 1911 and as late as the past few years. Some people had died in old age, but many more were young: twenties, thirties. On one section of the hillside, the graves belonged entirely to infants and children. A metal placard nearby read: *Dedicated to those whose lives and care we held in trust 'as seedlings of God we barely blossom on earth; we fully flower in Heaven.'* I felt very aware of my own body, then, my feet and ankles turning in underneath me, my contracting hamstrings and swollen knees, the steady pain radiating from my lower back into my toes. I remembered hearing about the doctor who told my parents, when I was born in 1991, that I would probably never live independently, might never even speak. I felt time and space collapse: sixty-five years ago, born in my hometown, I might have lived and died in the Colony, been buried in that field.

I went home that day and googled the Training Center under its old name. I read a little about Carrie Buck, the Colony inmate who'd been the named plaintiff in *Buck v. Bell,* the 1927 Supreme Court case that upheld Virginia sterilization laws and made eugenic sterilization legal throughout the United States. Forced to undergo compulsory sterilization after she was committed to the Colony while pregnant, Carrie was the perfect subject for testing the legal sturdiness of new sterilization statutes. She was declared the feebleminded daughter of a feebleminded mother, the first of three children with three different fathers. She and her family were the ideal lineage for eugenicists to cite when arguing that 'defectives' would overrun the population with their mental, physical, and moral flaws if they weren't kept forcibly and permanently in check.

When, in an 8-1 decision, the Supreme Court ruled it was in the state's interest to sterilize her, they legitimized the thousands and thousands of sterilizations that would follow—at the Colony and all over the country—and they underwrote the eugenicist philosophy on which Hitler would later base his "Law for the Prevention of Genetically

Diseased Offspring." When Oliver Wendell Holmes, Jr., then an Associate Justice, delivered the Court's famous ruling, he wrote: "Three generations of imbeciles are enough." Almost twenty years later, Nazi doctors at the Nuremberg Trials would cite that language as a defense. The Colony's history was a record of violence and discrimination that would radiate outwards, beyond national boundaries, for generations to come. It reverberated quietly inside my own life.

As seminal a case as Buck v. Bell was, there's remarkably little information from the years in the 1930s and 1940s at the height of the Colony's sterilization practices. Patient accounts are especially few and far between. In a regional newspaper story from the early 1990s, a Virginia reporter describes tracking down a former Colony patient who was released as a young woman and then spent her entire adult life trying to have children. Essentially, the reporter had to sit at the woman's kitchen table, look at her in her wheelchair, and tell her her own story: *This is what was done to you. This is the great shroud over your life, and you didn't even know about it.* Reading it, I wondered how the woman's face had altered then, if shock, or grief, or anger had bloomed first. I wondered if there was some relief in having even an awful explanation. There's a list of operations in my own life that helped make me who I am, but I have a record of every time a surgeon cut me open—the names of things that doctors declared wrong with me, the parts of me they've altered. I've lived my whole life with these catalogs. What would it be like to lack them? Or to have a stranger arrive one day at the home I'd made, bearing all that knowledge?

The virtual absence of patient accounts of Colony life during the eugenics movement is undoubtedly the result of a variety of forces: the lack of information inmates were given about their own histories and medical records; the pervasive sense that these "defective" people couldn't possibly have a meaningful perspective, an experience worth attending to, a complex and fully-realized inner life; and the amount of shame that surrounded being a former Colony resident, even after inmates were released. All these things collided to produce a history characterized as much by absence and silence as anything else.

Seeing the old pieces of the Colony, still standing there on the soil where I was raised, in the mountains I always recognized and claimed, even when the landscape of my own body felt foreign, tugged at me continually after my first visit to the grounds, but I wasn't ready to write about it immediately after passing through the gates. It would take me a few years to figure out how. And, though I didn't know it then, it would require reckoning not just with my proximity to the Colony and its history, but with the considerable space that shame and silence occupied in my own life.

A year after finishing college, I was living in Texas and teaching creative writing part-time to inner-city elementary school students. At twenty-one, I was an inexperienced teacher, and I struggled to control the kids in my classrooms. Released from the bounds of their usual school day, they leapt after one another between the aisles of their desks, moving faster than I could travel, into spaces where my wheelchair wouldn't fit. I felt unsuited for the work and, frankly, for life in the world. Most days, I came home in a lot of pain, with my knees and ankles swollen. My body resisted everything I asked of it, and I was tired, terrified, and furious.

My life was not going according to plan. Originally, I'd moved to Texas for graduate school, admitted straight out of undergrad to a prestigious writers' workshop. But I'd been unable to pass a required math class my senior year of college, or even a make-up course I'd taken online over the following summer. The same neurological damage that made my muscles spastic and my balance flawed also interrupted my ability to process numbers, space, and patterns. I'd gotten through high school math on a mix of hard work, charm, and the generosity of teachers who recognized my drive— but all my workarounds had limits. I was too ashamed to admit the degree to which I struggled, or to face the fact that I was flawed and damaged even beyond the boundaries of my body. I'd always been a gunner, foot on the gas and eyes on the horizon, ambitious about a future that promised to be better than whatever present I was in. I went to college at sixteen, and after two years, I left my tiny Massachusetts liberal arts school for a big California university and all the opportunities it held. My intellect, I'd taught myself early, was the one good part of me. Somewhere along the way, I developed the sense that if I were ambitious and extraordinary enough—if I did everything flawlessly and never stopped moving—I could outrun the truth of my body, leave it behind in the wake of all my excellence.

But no matter where I was, my brain fired stray signals across the same flawed circuit, my tendons pulled too tight, and my joints ached a little louder every year. I hurled myself from one city to another, one achievement to the next. But now the truth of my damage was intruding even on my mind. When, just a few weeks into my first semester of grad school, I found out that, even with tutoring, I hadn't done well enough on the final exam to pass the summer calculus course, I had to withdraw from the MFA program because I couldn't get a bachelor's degree immediately in hand.

Eventually, I got documentation to confirm my disability's cognitive effects and petitioned my university to wave the math requirement for my BA. I found the teaching job, restructured my life, but I no longer felt like I had any idea who I was. All the ways I understood myself—as smart, successful, useful—had been decimated, and everything I did felt animated by some combination of shame, and grief, and rage. The familiarity of the hills and valleys where I was raised had always been a source of steadiness in my life, and I turned toward trying to write about the Colony partly out of a reflexive impulse to return to that landscape. But I was also casting around for something that mattered: a way to contribute, to understand and articulate the histories of brains and bodies like mine. A way to face myself as I truly was.

I took a trip home to Virginia to drive again along the dusty gravel roads that threaded through the facility, to peer in the clouded window of the locked, low-slung Training Center chapel and look again at the tilted grid of grave markers covering the cemetery field. Back in Texas, I spent hours with the Image Archive on the American Eugenics Movement, pouring over scans of letters from eugenicist doctors and articles with titles like "The Burden of the Feebleminded" and "Freaks are Bred to Get New Knowledge of Heredity." I saved copies of black and white photographs of people labeled with diagnoses: *muscular atrophy, mania depressus, cretinism, spastic idiocy.* My own contemporary diagnosis is *spastic diplegia,* and I saw a subtle echo of the way I hold my own taut body in the curl of the boy seated on the stairs. Eventually, I found a blank copy of the sterilization order they would have used at the Virginia State Colony: a form headed *Before the State Hospital Board,* with a set of options available to indicate whether an inmate was *idiotic* or an *imbecile, feebleminded* or *epileptic.*

In the beginning, I had no idea what kind of project I was actually going to undertake. I'd done very little serious research before. But in the space left for an inmate's name on the sterilization order, I began to envision not just Carrie Buck's name, her mother Emma's, or her daughter Vivian's, but countless others: *Edith, Dorothy, Sarah, Addie, Marybeth, Caroline, Molly.* The more I learned, the less important and extraordinary my own individual pain seemed. Instead, the history from which my life extends came more sharply into focus: Much of the language I have for understanding my own body and brain is a permutation of vocabulary nurtured in the Colony. So many of the reasons I'd been running from myself stemmed from the same shame and fear, false equivalency and internalized ableism that enabled eugenicist thinking. So much of the life I've been able to lead is evidence of how far we've come from the height of the Colony's operations. So much of it is evidence of how far we still have to travel.

The more I learned about the Colony, the louder I began to hear a chorus of ghosts, the imagined voices of women in the Colony: women who were epileptic; women who were brilliant, but whose bodies left them unable to move or speak, and so who were assumed to be witless; women whose childhoods were stripped from them, who were never sent to school; women with their faces pressed to dormitory windows and their heads bowed in the modest chapel. I came home from teaching and wrote for hours, sitting on the couch with my legs propped up on pillows to ease the swelling. I ate handfuls of dry cereal out of the box because I didn't want to pause to make dinner. I fell asleep with every light in my house still on and the computer open and glowing.

In just a few months, I found I'd produced a claustrophobic little manuscript in the voices of these women, organized into the handful of rooms in which they would have lived, the ones I'd driven past and peered into while looping slow circles through Colony grounds. The poems were haunted, interior, and spare. I knew they couldn't stand in for the records of real patients' lives, but I hoped that they might be an act of kinship, that they would call attention to the devastating fact of all the thoughts, feelings, and discoveries that are lost to us because they happened inside the heads of women who were committed behind Colony walls, who were called *feeble* and *idiot* and *insane*, who were denied their right to be a part of society, to have a stake in the future of the world.

My own explicit presence in the manuscript remained only in a single opening poem, in which I narrated the trip through the Training Center's contemporary grounds and the circumstances that had brought me there. But the whole collection was shot through with my sense of how closely my body hewed to its history and landscape. I wanted my awareness that only an accident of time was responsible for the fact that I had *written* the poems in the book and not lived out one of the lives they detailed to open a door for the reader. And then I wanted to recede, and let a history I'd once known almost nothing of take center stage.

I wrote about the Colony when I had no choice but to sit still and live with my body and my brain, when I could no longer run from the fact of who I was. For a long time, without realizing it, I'd conceived of my disability only as a lack and a strangeness, a thing that divided me from my family and friends and most of the world. I'd avoided considering its contours any more intently than I had to to survive. I'd siphoned it off from the rest of me, like a tributary feeding into some far-off body of water. But the truth was, it tied me to a huge population of people who had lived before me, were living alongside me, and would come into the world once I had gone. And it emanated from this real shared heritage, made all the more devastating and complicated by the fact that so many Colony patients were denied the opportunity to have their own biological children, were bound together by the violence done to their bodies. Here was the truth of it, after all: I'd needed to grow smaller in my own imagination in order to know myself, to do the kind of work that really mattered. In order to realize I'd never, actually, been going it alone.

Calling Long Distance

There's SO MUCH standing at this party. Legs are the worst, I hate them! I send this text from the corner of my university's beginning-of-the-year department get-together, leaning heavily on my cane and trying to arrange my face in such a way that I don't look too uncomfortable. Our department chair's house is up two shallow flights of brick stairs, but even if I could get my wheelchair inside, the whole place is packed to the gills with people and I could never move in it. Instead, I make do relying on walls and various pieces of furniture for support. Periodically, I perch for a few minutes on the couch, but no one stays sitting long and, from down there, it's impossible to hear anyone who's standing due to the din. The expectation is that you'll circulate.

I love my colleagues, and I'm happy to see them, but every year I *hate* this party. There comes a point a little way into the evening when the pain in my knees, back, and ankles reaches a roaring point and my head is filled with the sound of a muffled ocean, as if my ear is pressed to the mouth of a conch shell. I can only half-concentrate on what anyone is saying to me. It's all muted, and my brain is busy balancing and breathing. Pain makes me tired. My body needs to rest, but it's more than that. I'm exhausted by feigning comfort, and I don't want to translate what's going on inside me, even for my friends. They're sorry when I'm hurting but, for them, the act of rising from the couch and standing is effortless and instant. The only thing that explaining my body will do is widen the gulf between us.

Usually, this is the point where I take myself off to the side for a moment and sit down apart from everyone. This year, though, my phone chimes quietly and brightly in my hand: *I was just thinking the same thing! THE WORST! Lots of standing here, too.* Susannah, another disabled poet, is texting from her own department party across the country, her ear pressed to her own roaring shell. Susannah and I publish with the same press, but, though we knew each other's work, we hadn't met until this summer when, by chance, we ended up at the same writer's conference. She found me the first night, and we fell in like we'd known one another forever, trading medical histories so extensive that one woman, shocked to overhear us, yelped, *You two are falling apart!* We laughed until we couldn't breathe. Since we've gone home to our separate states, we've spoken almost every day.

You're falling apart. This is a version of a truth I've known about myself ever since I can remember: *Your name is Molly.*

You have curly hair. You like to talk. You're falling apart. It's a part of the litany at the center of my self-conception. My particular type of CP increases my muscle tone and hinders my balance. I can walk—but only a little. I can stand—but not for long. My crouched, spastic gait puts too much pressure on my joints, and so the cartilage in my knees and ankles is wearing steadily away. I am, quite literally, falling apart, even if it is at a relatively gradual pace. This fact was delivered, first, in the mouths of doctors talking over my head to my parents about possible surgical and orthopedic interventions: *selective dorsal rhizotomy, partial hamstring release, heel cord lengthening, double-upright-KFOs.* Then I heard it from people who loved me, trying to give me the tools to live the rest of my life as painlessly and independently as possible, *I know it hurts, but you have to stretch, you have to walk, you have to put weight on your legs. Otherwise, you won't be able to walk anymore.* If you aren't walking, I learned, your body's no good. Somewhere along the way, I got cleaved down the middle. There was my damaged body, and then there was the rest of me, desperately trying to hold that body together, thinking: *I hate you*, and then, *I need you*, and then, *Thank you*, and then, *Please don't fall apart!*

These days, a lot of the language I use about my own life still reflects that split. I'm visibly disabled, and so I have to talk about my body everywhere I go. Sometimes it's to assuage people's curiosity. The woman in the shoe store wants to know what happened to me, or the man I'm on a first date with hasn't asked about my family but is transparently hungry for details about just what *exactly* my body can do, just how *exactly* I'm scarred. Sometimes explaining is a matter of necessity: I need to know if there's an elevator in the building where I teach this semester. Sometimes I'm not sure exactly why it is I'm explaining: On the first day of a new semester, I ask my students if they have any questions about me, and one boy puts up a hand and asks, utterly guileless: *So, what is it that's wrong with you?* I'm a relatively new teacher, and this hasn't happened to me before. Still, I answer him the way I've grown accustomed to answering. *I have a disability,* I say, like it's a shirt I put on in the morning. *It makes my balance bad. It means I don't walk very well.* After that, we have a conversation about why, in a writing class especially, being careful and exacting with our language is so important, but I can't stop that exchange from pinging around in my skull:

What is it that's wrong with you?

I have a disability.

The truth is that, even with the people who know and love me best, I have a nasty habit of treating my body like it's a bad suit of clothes or a thing that somehow just keeps *happening* to me. I don't talk much about it unless I need to explain: *I can't do this* or *could you give me a hand with that* or

I'm sorry, I can't go there. Mostly, I try to render it background noise. *Sometimes I forget you have a disability,* a friend says. A boyfriend said once, *It's such a small thing.* I did this on purpose. Their forgetting is my most impressive magic trick. Because I never forget about my disability, and the truth is, its root system is shot through every part of me. This is true on a basic biological level: It's a feature of my brain and the electrical signals it sends. But I mean it more deeply than that. It's not just that I'm often in pain, or that I have to think about my body almost all the time (although both these things are true). It's that I don't exist without my body. Its particular margins, movements, and methods for making it through the world are present, not just in the moments when it causes me hardship, but in the best and strongest stretches of my being. My body isn't standing apart from me holding my life in a vice grip. It is *making* my life, indivisible from the rest of me. We are walking together through the world, odd and slow as it looks.

I hate my legs, and I don't. I love my body, and I don't. There is a list of things that are wrong with me, and none of them are wrong with me. I go whole stretches of time without pausing to think, *I have a disability.* I am always, always, always disabled. When I make my life legible to an able-bodied world, all the nuance, all those contradictions, which aren't really contradictions, get sucked out of it, somehow.

Even I start to forget them. Any way you slice it, explaining is an act of erasure. Either I am describing my body so it can be understood and thereby forgotten (*look, it's not so scary after all—there it goes settling down in the corner to sleep*) or I am describing my body so that it begins to subsume the rest of me (*look, she grows curiouser and curiouser—that wheelchair, that weird walk, that way her hands curl up*).

Susannah and I are on the phone in the middle of a slow Tuesday, and I can't stop thinking how grateful I feel for her voice on the other end of the line. We're talking about our bodies, and then not about our bodies, about her dog, and my classes, and the zip line we'd like to string between us, from Mississippi all the way to Utah. And then we're talking about our bodies again, that sense of being both separate and not separate from the skin we're in. And it hits me all at once that none of this is in translation, none of this is explaining: *Legs are the worst,* I say, *I hate them.* And I know she knows I mean it, but that I also mean: *I love them.* And *I'm grateful* and *I'm glad you're here.* I also mean *I'm tired.* And I also mean *Thank God.*

Poetry, Patience, and Prayer

Recently, when the little liberal arts college in Virginia where they had taught for two decades appeared to be shutting its doors, my parents moved out of my childhood home on the campus to spend an uncertain year teaching at a boarding school in New England. Then, when the college's alumni rallied and it sputtered back to life, they returned to Virginia to be part of the school's second act. They did not, however, go back to the little clapboard farmhouse where I was raised. It stood empty during the year they were absent, falling apart without their tender attention. The gutter came loose from the roof, and a number of shingles were damaged. The doors and windows, already old and buckling, warped beyond easy repair. The back porch began to rot, its floorboards soft. My mother's beautiful garden went entirely to seed: all deer-munched weeds and groundhog tunnels, grass grown up beyond waist-height. We loved that house like a loyal, old dog. But my parents are edging toward sixty and, by the time they returned, it was beyond their ability or desire to salvage.

Instead, they moved into a newer home near the college's lake and began the process of unpacking all of their possessions on a new acre of the same landscape, situating their books, lamps, and chairs in whitewashed rooms less than a mile from where they'd stood before. My two siblings and I came back to help with the move at various points over the summer, each of us surprised to find an uncanny shadow version of our childhood waiting. The view of the mountains out the living room window was almost identical, but not quite. All our familiar furniture was in much the same configuration, with just a little more space around it. The ceilings were the same cool plaster but slightly higher, the floors the same oak boards, but without the warble when we walked. Even the light at twilight blued to the same shade, but beginning an instant later—I could swear it.

All of this had the effect of rendering everything we touched simultaneously foreign and familiar. Our childhood knickknacks waited in boxes for us to put them back where they belonged. As I unwrapped framed photographs slowly from dishtowels, I was surprised each time when the face of the child in the frame was mine. The distance between past and present ballooned and collapsed like a lung.

In the photo I paused over longest, I am eight years old and kneeling, eyes closed, in the great tiled hall of some European cathedral. My hands are clasped, and my chin is

tilted up towards the ceiling. Beside me, a doll lies abandoned. This photo is misleading for a number of reasons. It
suggests a youth full of glamorous international travel when,
in fact, aside from this one extraordinary trip to Europe when
my father was on sabbatical, I've still never been outside the
country. More than that, though, looking at the picture, you'd
think I was a peaceful, patient, pious child, the kind of girl
about whom people are always saying, *She's so well behaved,
she's so sweet, look at her manners.*

In reality, nothing could be further from the truth. I was
a wild, dramatic, emotional kid, messy and loud, demanding
and impatient. And really, I shouldn't talk in the past tense—
I'm still so many of these things. My childhood was marked
and measured by a host of interventions intended to address
the effects of neurological disorder that heightens my muscle
tone and hinders my balance. For years I cycled between the
hospital, the orthopedist's office, and physical therapy. I had
multiple surgeries, wore huge plaster casts, metal knee immo-
bilizers that thatched the backs of my thighs with lacerations,
and more types of leg braces than I can count. I spent a lot of
time in waiting rooms. My parents woke me before the sun
was up to do the same routine of small, miserable exercises
every morning. In the evenings, we did them again. Hours of
our lives disappeared this way. Everything about the repetition, discipline, and slowness that my life required made me

furious. I wanted to run, to leap, to burst out of my own body and then beat it to a pulp. I was a badly built machine, and almost nothing came easily. The one thing, in fact, that I have ever felt meant for, or made for, in any sense—and from my earliest moments—is poetry.

My family is not religious. While I was raised in the epicenter of fundamentalist Southern Baptism, our little academic enclave didn't have much use for God. Instead, we were readers. My parents are writers, too, and while there wasn't any scripture in our living room, I grew up on my father reading us Walker Percy and Flannery O'Connor and Walt Whitman, ecstatic and electric, or my mother reading C. S. Lewis, quoting Richard Wilbur's "Love Calls Us to the Things of the World," and Gerard Manley Hopkins' "Pied Beauty." All those dappled things: *original, spare, strange.* I can remember discovering my mother's copy of Emily Dickinson's poems at maybe seven or eight years old and, of course, not really understanding any of it, but reading: *The soul has moments of escape—/ When bursting all the doors—/ She dances like a Bomb, abroad,* and feeling the music, the strangeness, and the desperate compression of it. I can remember thinking: *That. I want to do that.* Knowing, somehow, that she was worrying that difficult space between body and soul.

In my daily life, I was desperate to wrench away from my body, and I hated how stumblingly and ploddingly it moved, but in poetry I found a form that not only mirrored my own slowness, but rewarded the careful attention with which I had to move through the world. *Things / that can't move / learn to see*, writes poet Louise Glück in "The Hawthorne Tree." *I do not need to chase you through the garden.* If there's a refrain for my poetic existence, this is it: poetry as the place in which slowness, repetition, necessary stillness become the territory of potential, and understanding, and even transcendence.

I don't mean to suggest that, once I found my way to poetry, I transformed into the peaceful, prayerful child kneeling on the floor of that cathedral, or to argue that the move from a love for poetry into a place of religious faith is either linear or inevitable. I do know, though, that for me, poetry and faith are both—most centrally—a matter of attending to the world: of slowing my pace, and focusing my gaze, and quieting my impatient, indignant, protesting heart long enough for the hard shell of the ordinary to break open and reveal the stranger, subtler singing underneath.

Christian Wiman has a poem that I love called "Every Riven Thing." It goes:

God goes, belonging to every riven thing he's made
sing his being simply by being
the thing it is:

stone and tree and sky,
man who sees and sings and wonders why

God goes. Belonging, to every riven thing he's made,
means a storm of peace.
Think of the atoms inside the stone.
Think of the man who sits alone
trying to will himself into a stillness where

God goes belonging. To every riven thing he's made
there is given one shade
shaped exactly to the thing itself:
under the tree a darker tree;
under the man the only man to see

God goes belonging to every riven thing. He's made
the things that bring him near,
made the mind that makes him go.
A part of what man knows,
apart from what man knows,

God goes belonging to every riven thing he's made.

Each time I read this poem, I am swallowed by the sound
of it, and struck all over again by the way it enacts its own

prayerfulness, that initial phrase, *God goes belonging to every riven thing he's made,* repeating and shifting to admit music and loneliness, doubt and desire before it arrives back at itself at the poem's end. The whole engine of the poem is sustained attention to this one unit of language, which, as it is revisited, insists that stillness is *difficult* work we have to will ourselves into: admitting a God who is present even in our inability to find him. The word I can't get over here is *riven:* split, severed, torn apart. When we will ourselves to stillness, we find we are flawed and cleaved inherently. A rip is a wound that might undo you, but also a space where light comes through.

This idea that being riven is a state of grace and potential matters to me especially acutely. The scars on my legs and back are evidence of the ways I have been literally split. And, at the core of me, there is a permanent gash where my twin sister and I were once joined. One single egg split into two of us, and in her dying, we were split again. I feel the canyon in me, where she should be, all the time: a loss prior to memory. Each of my beginnings is a tearing. Ripped. Rent. Riven. So often, I am trying to rush myself away from the truth of that.

And so I don't find this labor of stilling myself for either God or poetry to be especially gentle work. More often than not, I go to the desk, or to Mass, resisting all the way. John Donne writes:

BATTER my heart, three person'd God; for, you
As yet but knocke, breathe, shine, and seeke to mend;
That I may rise, and stand, o'erthrow me, and bend
Your force, to breake, blowe, burn and make me new

To write—or to pray—I have to give myself up to the battering. I am as impatient, and demanding, and sometimes furious as I ever was. Most often, I quiet and close my eyes and attend only when the world gives me no other option. But when I yield to it, stillness is always a place of discovery. *Think of the atoms inside a stone.* The infinite collides with the infinitesimal. I get a poem. I get a palpable sense of God.

In an interview about theology and poetry, Fanny Howe says: *Half of me every day wakes up and feels alien, alienated on a dangerous planet.* But there is something, she says, *in our material bodies that protects itself around an organizing principle . . . if you turn in and draw on that principle you can save yourself.* That's the principle of poetry, she insists. It's like *unifying your soul, integrating your being in spite of everything that's being taken away from you.* Through it, she's found, you can save yourself.

Perhaps it seems odd for someone with such a fraught relationship to her corporeal body to find comfort in Howe's notion that something in poetry is tied to our physical selves, and that—through it—we can engender some harmony between our bodies and our souls, some sense of cohesion in our being. But if poetry is the territory of stillness, and the singing, straining, riven thing, then it's the territory in which I know how to make sense of the margins of my body—and the manner in which it works its way through the world. I was *built* to slow and pay attention. When I yield, consent, and do it, something in me harmonizes. Call it what you will: purpose, grace, *a storm of peace.*

God goes belonging to every riven thing he's made.

THE BROKEN COUNTRY:
ON DISABILITY AND DESIRE

The fall I was nineteen, I came into my college dining hall in California just in time to overhear a boy telling a table of our mutual acquaintances that he thought I was very nice, but he felt terribly sorry for me because I was going to die a virgin. This was already impossible, but in that moment all that mattered was the blunt force of the boy's certainty. He hadn't said, *I could never . . .* or, *She might be pretty but . . .* or, *Can she even have sex?* or even, *I'd never fuck a cripple,* all sentences I'd heard or overheard by then. What he had done was, firmly, with some weird, wrong breed of kindness in his voice, drawn a border between my body and the country of desire.

It didn't matter that, by then, I'd already done my share of heated fumbling in narrow dorm room beds then going home in the early light in last night's clothes; that more than one person had already looked at me and said, *I'm in love with you,* and I had said it back. It didn't matter that I'd boldly kissed a boy on his back porch in sixth grade, surprising him so much that the BB gun he was holding went off and sent a squadron of brown squirrels skittering up into the trees. Most of me was certain that the boy in the dining hall was right in all the ways that really mattered. He knew I'd never be the kind of woman anyone could really want, and I knew that even my body's own wanting was suspect and tainted by flaw. My body was a country of error and pain. It was a doctor's best attempt, a thing to manage and make up for. It was a place to leave if I was hunting goodness, happiness, or release.

*

I have the strongest startle reflex in the world. Call my name in the quiet, make a loud noise, introduce something sudden into my field of vision, and I'll jump like there's been a clap of thunder every time. It's worst, though, if you touch me when I'm not expecting it. I start the way an animal does, frightened and feral. For years, I thought only the bad wiring in my brain was to blame, the same warped signals that throw off my balance and make my muscles tighten, keeping me permanently on tenterhooks. Then I met Susannah, whose first memories are also a gas mask, and a surgeon's hands: being picked up, held down, put under. She, too, jumps at the smallest surprise, the slightest unanticipated touch. Now, I think it's also something in that early trauma: all those years of being touched without permission, having your body handled and talked about over your head, being forced to slip between waking and sleeping, to leave your body and come back to a version that hurts more, but is supposedly better—the blank stretch of time that's just emptiness, when something happened you can't name. I think it matters that the first touch I remember is someone readying to cut me open. That when I woke up, I was crying, and there was a sutured wound.

*

For the better part of my childhood, I was part of a study on gait development in children with cerebral palsy. What this means is that, at least once a year—and sometimes more frequently, if I'd had recent surgery—I spent an afternoon in a research lab, walking up and down a narrow strip of carpet, with sensors and wires attached to my body so doctors could chart the way I moved. The digital sensors compiled a computer model of my staggering shape, each one a little point of light, and when I peeled them off, they left behind burning red squares like perfect territories. But the doctors also shot the whole thing on a video camera, mounted on a tripod, and gave us the raw footage to take home. The early films are cute: I'm curly-haired and chatty. The bathing suit I wear so that my legs and arms are bare is always either a little too small or a little too big, a hand-me-down from my older sister. I trundle happily down the carpet. As I get older, though, the tapes get more complicated. By the time I get to footage where I look anything like myself, I can't bear to watch it anymore. I'm a teenage girl in bike shorts or a bathing suit, being watched by a collection of men, walking what's essentially a runway like some kind of staggering, wounded animal.

Even today, I can't quite tell: Do I hope that when they looked at me back then, mostly undressed, they saw only a crop of defects that needed fixing, a collection of their best repairs? Or do I hope that one of them—maybe the redhead, not yet thirty—felt some small press of desire, knew I was a girl on the edge of womanhood and not a half-lame horse or subject #53? I know I hated being watched. I also know it never occurred to me that anyone watching would see something worth wanting. They took those videos through most of my adolescence. Do you know I still can't stand to watch myself walk? I put my eyes on the floor when I pass department store mirrors, or a window's reflective glass. I catch a glimpse of myself and my stomach turns. When I asked the first man that I loved about the way I moved he said, *It's nothing. It doesn't matter*—he meant it as a comfort—but I thought, *You're wrong. It makes me what I am.*

*

Chronic pain makes you good at abandoning yourself. It teaches you that your body is a thing to ignore until it insists on being noticed—until your joints ache too badly to stand, until something buckles, until you fall and then you're bleeding hard enough to stain your clothes. There's a certain low thrum of hurt I don't notice; it's just the frequency at the bottom of everything, my version of the ground. A good day is one where I hardly think about my body, where I adjust for its flaws by instinct, where there isn't any sudden spike in that low pulse of pain.

On a good day, my body doesn't embarrass me. It does what I ask it. I don't notice people staring, don't trip on my way in to teach a class and send thirty-five student papers flying everywhere. I don't have to pause at a threshold and ask a stranger to help me lift my wheelchair up and though a door. No one I don't really know needs to put their hands on me. No one in the grocery store asks, *What happened, sweetie? You're so pretty to be in a wheelchair!* On a good day, my body pulls hard at the hem of my dress, and I hiss back, *You don't exist,* and it goes somewhere else, or I do.

In bed, a man pauses, puts a wide, gentle hand on my face and asks: *Honey, where are you? Come back here.* I want to, and also I don't.

*

Just as I hit adolescence, my body abruptly began to break down. I grew, and so did my physical instability. My tendons tightened, and my pain increased. The doctors scheduled another set of medical procedures: a surgery, a summer in a set of full-leg plaster casts, a pair of heavy, bulky metal braces. Just as I began to learn I could feel sexual desire, I was splintered and in pain again, and the fact of it demanded most of my attention. My earliest experiences with lust feel shrunken by the trauma: vague and distanced, like I watched through a scratched viewfinder as they happened to someone else. I can't identify them for you except as strange, dark shapes at an unreachable horizon line.

Those years, I had to wear parachute pants—specially made by a tailor who regularly asked my mother to remind her what was wrong with me—and giant sneakers to accommodate the braces. Besides all that, I had the usual adolescent problems: hadn't learned that you really just shouldn't brush curly hair, or that if you have hips and spend most of your time sitting or bent over, low-rise jeans are a terrible idea. Not only was I far from resembling the kind of girl I could imagine anyone finding desirable, I was so occupied with pain and with being a patient, perpetually hamstrung between being taken apart and put back together, that it would take me years to really look at myself and realize, *Oh, I'm also a person. A woman. There's a whole other way I can want to be touched.*

I belonged to an adaptive skiing association and spent most of the time I wasn't in the hospital or physical therapy learning to hurl myself down snow-covered mountains with men who'd been paralyzed in car wrecks. But I didn't know a single adult woman with a disability really comparable to mine. Nowhere on television, or in any magazine, did I see any portrayals of disabled women as sexual and desirable (let alone as partners or as parents), and most of the solace the early 2000s internet had to offer me was in the form of assurance that I might one day be the object of some very particular fetish. It matters that, when any adult spoke to me about my body, they did so in purely utilitarian terms, said that I should want the best range of motion, the least pain, the highest level of mobility, so that I could one day buy groceries, live independently, hold a job. Of course, nobody warned: *You'll want your hamstrings to be loose enough that it doesn't hurt when your muscles tense before you have an orgasm.* They also didn't say: *We want to do all this to you so that one day your body can be a thing that brings you pleasure, a thing that you don't hate.*

The truth is my first real flushes of lust, of that sudden carnal pull toward another body, happened when my *own* body was a dangerous thing, one I couldn't trust not to fall to pieces or to lunge at the rest of me with its teeth bared, out for blood. So much of my somatic experience was agonizing and frightening. I had no idea what my body would look, move, or feel like five years down the line. Desire wasn't entirely crowded out by pain, but I distrusted it the same way I did everything that felt born in my body: as if it was an instant away from morphing into suffering, waiting only until I attended to it to become a thing that hurt me. I playacted at desire often—mimicking the adolescents around me when they traded gossip about crushes, had first kisses, held hands furtively underneath their desks in social studies class—but I couldn't afford to get to know its real contours in my life, to attend to my own sensations, or to believe in a future that had real space for that kind of pleasure or intimacy, that kind of love. To survive, I had to stay unfamiliar to myself, neutralized, at arm's length. Sometimes, I think, all these years later, I'm still hunting the part of myself I exiled.

When I was newly seventeen, a beautiful girl I loved put her head in my lap, said, *You're so gorgeous,* and then leaned up and kissed me. I would spend the better part of the next year alternately pushing her away and pulling her close, trying to figure out whether I wanted her, too, or only the plain unapologetic fact of her desire for me. Her gentleness, her confidence in her own body and its hunger, the fact that, when she watched me move, I felt like a painting come to life and not a patient or a busted wind-up toy. A decade later, I still feel guilty for all the secretive back-and-forth I put her through, and the answer to that question still feels fraught and muddy.

A handful of years after that, I was in a coffee shop with a man I half-thought I'd marry, in a youthful abstract way, and someone in line assumed he was my brother, though we could not look less alike. When we corrected her, she looked over my head at him and said, voice gentle and admiring,

She's so lucky to have found you. He bit his tongue when I squeezed his hand. I didn't want to think about it anymore. We turned away.

We started dating after he came to a reading I gave. When it was over, he came up and kissed my cheek, said, *That was so beautiful that I forgot to breathe while you were talking,* then turned on his heel and walked away. I rolled my eyes, thought, *God, I can't believe he really tried that line,* but couldn't get him out of my head. The way I moved was nothing, he was proof it didn't matter.

At a taffy shop on the boardwalk in San Francisco the weekend we first say, *I love you,* a middle-aged man is pushing a woman, clearly his wife, in a wheelchair. They are laughing, and his head is bent so that their faces are close together as he walks, intimate and tender. We collide in the aisle and pause—two couples smiling at one another—while we make room for her wheelchair to get past mine. They walk on, and then we kiss, fierce and happy there. We don't know anything. We both think *maybe.*

Later, we're in Florida at the beach, and I've been stiff and hurting for weeks from a summer of travel. In the bathroom, while we're changing into bathing suits, he looks me up and down. I'm prepared for him to try something—to kiss me—and I'm prepared to put him off, we don't have time; we have to meet my family by the water. Instead, he asks me tenderly,

Do you want help clipping your toenails, baby? They're getting kind of long. That night, in bed, I roll away when he reaches for me. My body is no country for desire.

A couple of years later still, another man—charming, boy-next-door beautiful, and quarterback confident—has started spending evenings in my bed, or with me pinned to his couch. He tells me I'm beautiful, asks to read what I'm writing, then asks quiet questions about poetry and movies that I love. But he won't be seen dating me in public. When I tell him I'm *more* than happy to be fooling around, but that I won't sleep with somebody I hardly know, he puts all his weight on top of me, says, *Oh, if I wanted to have sex with you, you'd know.* Then flips me over. Pushes my head down hard enough that it hurts. I think, *He's embarrassed to be seen with me. He gets off on how fragile I am. I'm too old to put up with this.* But I let him. I let it go on for weeks and weeks like that.

Always, I'm aware that I'm particularly vulnerable. I couldn't run if you came at me. I'd fall to the ground if you touched me even slightly roughly. No balance. No steadiness. I will always start at an unexpected hand.

*

But because some of you are wondering (I see you leering at me, stranger at the bank. I see you, terrible internet date); because we live in the world we do, a world that often assumes disabled people are sexless or infantile; because I wish I had heard anyone who looked or moved like me say it when I was fourteen; I want to be very clear: I *can,* in fact, have sex. I am a woman who *wants* in ways that are both abstract and concrete. I have turned down advances from people I wasn't attracted to, and said *yes* to a few advances I'm sorry about now, and more that have been lovely, surprising, and good. I've had a date who didn't realize I was in a wheelchair turn and walk out of a restaurant when he saw me, and I've watched the light behind men's eyes turn from desire to curiosity to something else when they realize something's *wrong with me.* I've been hit on while on barstools by people who disappear once they've watched me get up and shuffle slowly to the bathroom. I've used that trick to my advantage. I've spent a stormy weekend taking baths and eating overripe peaches in a seedy motel with someone I loved, and another getting lusty-whiskey-drunk with someone I didn't, but whom I was still perfectly happy to have unbutton my shirt. The finer points I'll keep to myself, except to say that my familiarity with how to jump-rope the line between pleasure and pain has done me some favors. If you're listening, younger self, some of what you're learning will eventually have uses no one's naming for you now, I swear.

*

If this were a different kind of essay, I would leave it there. Or I would tell you that I've arrived at a reconciled point: that no part of me ever still believes that the boy in the dining hall, who was certain I would die a virgin, hit on some real truth about the ways my body is defective and repellent; that, now, I can watch myself move without feeling some small wave of shame; that I've completely stopped abandoning my body out of instinct, or habit, or what feels like necessity, in moments when it should bring me pleasure and intimacy and joy. I would tell you that I've fully worked out how to have a partner who I know really sees my body, its contours, its scars and its pain, who I can let give me the particular kinds of help I need and still trust sees me as sexual and desirable. But this isn't that kind of story. I don't know exactly where the reconciled point is, or even what it looks like.

Instead, things just get more complicated. I really want children and, in the last few years, that prospect has collided with these questions of intimacy and desire. I worry about finding a partner truly willing to parent with me in the ways I know my disability will necessitate, and to sign up for the medical uncertainties I know are around the bend in my own life. I worry about the toll pregnancy might take on my body, and about being physically capable of being a good parent once my children are born. I worry that my clock is ticking faster than most people's, my body wearing down and wearing out. And, in the hardest moments, that whatever small kind of beauty and desirability I might, in fact, possess is wearing away with it. I'm still surprised by my own limits, still frustrated and exhausted by pain. Sometimes I still feel suspicious of all my body's sensations, the good ones snarled too completely with the bad. But not all moments are the hardest ones, and maybe the point is simply this: that I am still alive, still in the business of heading *somewhere,* still a woman who can stumble, hurt, and want, and—yes—be wanted. That there is no perfect reconciliation, only the way I hold it all suspended: wonderful, and hugely difficult, and true.

The Cost of Certainty

On three acres, near the top of Candlers Mountain in Lynchburg, Virginia, there's a wide clear-cut space. Where trees once stood, white gravel has been poured in a perfect circle over the clay. In the center, low shrubs flanked by dark maroon pebbles form the letters LU. It's called the Mountain Top Monogram, and you can see it from the highway, from the nearby shopping center, from most of the city below. You can see it for miles. LU stands for Liberty University. Founded by the Reverend Jerry Falwell in 1971 as Lynchburg Baptist College, the school now bills itself as the world's largest Christian university, its motto *Training Champions for Christ*. In practice, this means that Liberty has more than fourteen thousand residential students on a seven-thousand-acre campus and another nearly hundred-thousand students enrolled in more than two hundred-eighty online programs. It has a law school, a college of osteopathic medicine, and, of course, a divinity school. It has a ski slope (covered year-round in Snowflex synthetic snow), more than fifty miles of dedicated trail space, a skating rink, and a movie theater. By every metric, Liberty is vast and steadily expanding. Expansion is part of the point. The school's doctrinal statement affirms that religious institutions are responsible for *carry[ing] out the commission to evangelize, to teach, and to administer the ordinances of believer's baptism and the Lord's table.* To spread the word of God, you have to grow.

*

I grew up on the campus of a little, secular women's college about twenty-five miles north of Lynchburg. My parents are English professors, and my family is not a churchgoing one. My father has a Louisiana ex-Catholic boy's love of saints and all their strangeness, and my mother has impeccable manners and a Protestant work ethic that never exhausts itself—but that's about as far as they go with religion. In our household, Liberty was shorthand for a particular brand of Fundamentalist Southern Baptism, heavy on bigotry and brimstone and short on nuance, intellect, and kindness. When the university razed the side of Candlers Mountain to install their logo in 2007, we were horrified at what we saw—frankly, what I still see—as the narcissism and lack of environmental responsibility inherent in the gesture. When I told my mother on the phone that I was planning to open this essay with a description of the monogram, she sighed audibly. *That thing*, she said, *will be there forever.*

There wasn't much to do in my one-stoplight hometown, and in junior high, I spent a lot of afternoons in the Lynchburg Barnes & Noble, where the Christian literature selection dwarfed the poetry shelf and the YA section bulged with dystopic series set in the aftermath of the Rapture. Liberty students hung around the bookstore cafe with notebooks and laptops or loafed in the overstuffed armchairs near the back. Sometimes, we made trivial conversation. They'd bend their heads at me in the manner of teenagers being kind to slightly younger kids, and ask my name and whether I was from around there. Eventually, the conversation would almost always make its way around to a question about where my family went to church, and they'd look genuinely sad when I told them we didn't. Mostly, it never went much beyond that. They'd tell me I could come to Thomas Road Baptist Church anytime, and then I'd drift back to whatever trashy novel about a maladjusted teenager dying of cancer I was currently reading in the aisle between bookshelves.

Once, though, a girl with an eyebrow piercing that matches one I have now, fifteen years later, kept me talking a beat longer. She bent down until our faces were level, put a hand on my wheelchair tire, and told me that I really ought to come to church. *It'll heal your pain,* she said, her voice sure and imploring. I don't remember what I did then. Probably I made some noncommittal noise and moved away to another corner of the store. I didn't know whether the healing she spoke about was physical or only emotional and spiritual, but I knew that, regardless, she saw something she thought needed healing in my disabled body. I'd already developed enough of a political consciousness to call that ableism, and I'd had enough experience with people who saw me as damaged to feel indignant and hurt. However, in that moment, I was also jealous of her certainty, which, when she held her face close to mine, felt so present and constant I could nearly touch it. She knew what mattered. Where to go for comfort and for steadying. The God she believed in was knowable and reachable. A force that healed.

It is this sense of palpable certainty and comfort that I still find magnetic in the Evangelical faith, even as I bristle at the politics that typically accompany it. To evangelize requires a level of conviction and assurance I envied as a teenager, and sometimes still catch myself yearning for now. I spent a good part of my early years ricocheting between the hospital and the physical therapist's office: one surgery, or casting procedure, or set of heavy plastic leg braces after another, all designed to try and correct the damage done by a neurological disorder that causes my muscles to contract constantly, setting me perpetually off balance. For years, I clunked around in various unwieldy orthopedic contraptions, moved slowly, repeated the same rote, painful exercises: Lift your leg two inches off the ground, and lay it down again. Again. Again. In a different world, this kind of meditative work would have been the thing to teach me equanimity. Instead, all it did was infuriate me and engender a rabid desire to do more, to move faster, to spill out over the bounds of my own body—outrun it, leave it behind. After surgery, I'd shut myself in my room for hours until I learned to dress myself again. Lock the door so no one could come in to help. I beat the hell out of a punching bag in the child psychiatrist's office. I wailed. I wanted what I wanted, and I wanted it now: a cookie, a dog, a different body. I did not come easily or gently to anything: not to patience, or devotion, or gratitude, or the thing I have learned to call faith. Everything about my world shook.

*

Jerry Falwell was only twenty-two when, in 1956, he founded Thomas Road Baptist Church in his hometown of Lynchburg. Falwell's father and grandfather weren't churchgoers. In fact, his grandfather was a vocal atheist. But his mother's unwavering belief seems to have been enough to bring him to God. Writers love to quote a line in Falwell's autobiography about getting saved as a teenager: *I accepted the mystery of God's salvation. I didn't doubt it then. I haven't doubted it to this day.* According to an old church pamphlet, Falwell, who once aspired to a professional baseball career, *rejected the call of the St. Louis Cardinals and accepted the call of God*; he went to Baptist Bible College in Missouri and then came home to start his thirty-five-member church. He had an instinct for evangelizing, and he immediately began to broadcast his sermons on a radio program called *The Old-Time Gospel Hour*. Within six months, they were also being broadcast on local Virginia television.

Falwell died in 2007, and his church now has more than twenty-four thousand members. His television program has gone into international syndication, and you can stream the sermons his son Jonathan gives straight from the church's website. The main sanctuary looks like an arena. It has stadium seating, and the stage that holds the pulpit is outfitted for light shows and concerts. The church has satellite campuses in the nearby cities of Danville and Roanoke, as well as an entirely separate chapel where services are conducted in Spanish. There's a reason they call it a megachurch. Falwell's certainty has built a ministry on the scale of the God it champions, the God of Jeremiah 33:3, who answers the believers who call to him and shows them *great and mighty things* they did not know before.

Thomas Road Baptist, Liberty University, and Liberty Christian Academy, a K–12 day school founded in the 1960s, form a kind of trinity, the three pillars of an Evangelical ministry in Lynchburg. One proceeds from the other like the Holy Spirit from the Son, and the Son from the Father, all three *one in essence but distinct in person and function.* Each piece runs separately but is designed to rear, shape, and eventually sustain generations of Evangelicals whose belief is as stable as the institutions themselves and who become engines of the church's expansion, raising their children in what the faith calls a *culture of prayer* and a *lifestyle of worship* with a *passion for sharing* designed to reach the *uttermost parts of the earth.* Marketing materials from both Liberty and Thomas Road Baptist Church quote Romans 10:14: *How then shall they call on Him in whom they have not believed? And how shall they believe in Him of whom they have not heard? And how shall they hear without a preacher?* Believers must be committed, they remind you, to *intentionally developing relationships that 'earn'. . . the right to actively share the Gospel.*

For Falwell, this commitment to spreading the word of God always went beyond religion; it was explicitly cultural and political. In 1979, he founded the Moral Majority, an organization designed to mobilize the Christian Right, and Evangelical voters specifically, to influence American politics. The issues on which they campaigned, as much as they were in some sense indicative of the political landscape in the 1980s, will look familiar to anyone paying attention to politics today. They promoted what they called a *traditional version of family life,* which meant opposing any state recognition of *homosexual acts,* advocating for the prohibition of abortion even in cases of rape and incest, and opposing the Equal Rights Amendment. Structured to tackle issues on local, state, and national levels, they advocated for Christian prayer in public schools and financially backed initiatives designed to market conservative Christianity to nonbelievers. Though the Moral Majority would formally dissolve before 1990, Falwell never really gave up its aims, and a few years before his death, he revived it, this time calling it the Moral Majority Coalition, its central objectives and oppositions much the same.

Certainty has an ugly side. Although he'd recant the view in later years, in the 1950s and '60s Jerry Falwell was an unapologetic segregationist, and Liberty Christian Academy was initially formed in response to court-mandated integration; the student body is still overwhelmingly white. Falwell was known for his venomous anti-gay tirades, and the version of America he sought, both spiritually and politically, was designed to make little room for anyone who didn't think exactly like him.

But what has always interested me about Falwell and his many disciples is a phenomenon the journalist Kevin Roose describes in his 2009 book *The Unlikely Disciple* about his experience of enrolling as a student at Liberty despite not being a believer. *I honestly think he believes every word he preaches*, Roose writes of Falwell, *and I wouldn't be at all surprised if he really does stay awake at night worrying about the homosexual agenda, the evils of abortion and the imminent spread of liberalism. He really does think America needs to be saved.*

From my own position in the world, the politics Falwell espoused, and the ones his son Jerry Falwell Jr. continues to trumpet now as president of Liberty University, are repugnant and clearly damaging in their unyielding-ness, in their judgment, in the narrow kind of life they seem willing to sanction as beautiful, useful, or good. But what do we do with the fact that, at least in some measure, these politics arise out of a real wellspring of conviction: a love for the God you know has saved you, and a fervent fear that every man and woman you don't manage to reach is lost to that grace? Falwell's Evangelicalism asserts that *the return of Christ for all believers is imminent* and that, when it happens, *the saved, having been raised, will live forever in heaven in fellowship with God.* The unsaved will be *judged according to their works and separated forever from God in hell.* Falwell wouldn't have called his beliefs (political or otherwise) judgmental. Judgment is the territory of God. But what else are you to do but be unyielding when the eternal fate of every nonbeliever rests on your shoulders?

Much has been written, some of it quite compellingly, by outsiders like Roose *infiltrating* Liberty to paint a picture of Evangelical America, its leaders and its youth. And perhaps even more has been made, in recent years, of Jerry Falwell Jr.'s early, vocal support of Donald Trump, who spoke at Liberty's forty-fourth commencement in May 2017. But, if I'm telling the truth, these kinds of tell-alls about Evangelical America don't interest me much, nor does Falwell Jr.'s insistent endorsement of the president's agenda. Because Trump's behavior so blatantly conflicts with biblical teaching, Falwell Jr.'s support just feels to me like complicity in the service of power and of his own business interests as Liberty expands. Their political marriage seems clearly rooted not in faith, but in pragmatism: the polar opposite of Evangelicalism's necessarily uncompromising moral certainty, and the God it insists is real.

I've struggled mightily with my own belief in God, and with its accompanying relationship to religious institutions, and so I *am* interested in how those at Liberty do, or don't, make their peace with Trump, and with Falwell's vocal support of him. How their faith—their certainty—plays into this. Evangelicals may be certain of what perfection looks like, but we all have to make our way forward in an imperfect world.

*

This is where I tell you that, in graduate school, after many years of resisting my own faith, of flitting between church services from many denominations, and of attending Mass without fully participating or speaking to anyone, I converted to Catholicism. The truth is that I believe, with a fierceness I can't quantify, and in a way I have no articulate explanation for, that people have souls, that none of us is an accident, and that we are not unattended or alone. I believe that we're all cleft from something greater than ourselves. This notion— that being cleft can be a kind of gift—has a particular urgency for me, both as someone whose body has been literally rent and re-sewn again and again by the gloved hands of surgeons working at her stubborn muscles and her bowing bones, and as someone whose identical twin died when we were infants, too small to outlast our early, hurried coming. My body is mapped with visible scars, and the thing I've learned to call my soul has a raw, ragged margin where I was once tethered to my sister. I miss her with the kind of vague, omnipresent ache you can only have for something you have known exclusively as absence, but also with an intense specificity that has no rational cause.

So much about my faith is mysterious to me, and all I know is that, when I participate in Mass, I feel like a better version of myself. Closer to God and closer to whole. The ground steadies underneath my feet. Most strict Catholics would call me a Cafeteria Catholic: content to accept the parts of the theology and the liturgy that are important to me, while leaving off my tray the parts of the Church's politics that don't always cleanly align with my own convictions. And it's true that I go to Mass and I take Communion while supporting gay marriage and advocating for reproductive rights—certain that life inside the womb is real from its earliest beginnings, and also that we have no business legislating abortion when there are all kinds of deeply complex reasons, both individual and systemic, that someone might not be able or ready or willing to be a mother, or even to carry a child. I've made my peace with the tensions there, even when they aren't easy. I call myself a Catholic, and mean it, both when I'm proud of the Church and when I'm embarrassed by it. I believe in the God at the heart of it, even when I quarrel with the way people interpret the theology or want to carry it out. It's also true that, lately, I haven't wanted to go to church. I've been hollowed out and uselessly furious at all the people using Christianity as some kind of excuse for hatred, abuse, and rabid fear-mongering; pretending all faith doesn't have a deep and essential common denominator; ignoring the fact that the scripture they profess to hold so sacred models over and over again just how essential it is to welcome the stranger, embrace the foreigner, feed the hungry, and be a force for justice and peace.

I've written a little about my faith, but my language for it is still nebulous and inchoate, my hold on it still new. And, often, in the last year, I confess it has felt all but gone. I haven't known what to pray for, felt much beyond a void. Sometimes I go to Mass only out of some faint muscle-memory and the sense that, if I don't, I'll just sit in my apartment scrolling through headlines. Part of what I'm hunting, in my inquiry about Liberty and Evangelicalism, is some sort of understanding of how to hold on to your certain faith even when the way it's put into practice feels damningly human and flawed.

*

In August, *Mother Jones* published an article about a coalition of Liberty alumni organizing to return their diplomas in protest of Falwell Jr.'s support of Trump, which held steadfast even during the bipartisan backlash in response to his egregious comments after the white supremacist rally in Charlottesville last summer. A young alumna told reporter Becca Andrews that Trump's behavior was *beyond the pale*, and that a *Christian university is called to be morally correct and ethically correct, to show kindness to the hurting, and to condemn wrongdoing where necessary.* These outraged Liberty alumni still identify as Christians, even Evangelicals, but they no longer want to claim an affiliation with Liberty as long as Falwell Jr. claims an affiliation with Trump.

This sort of distancing is rare; more than eighty percent of Evangelicals voted for Trump in the 2016 election. In the voting precinct on Liberty's campus, that number was almost eighty-five percent. When I ask Karen Swallow Prior, who teaches English at Liberty, if she thinks this number is indicative of students' widespread excitement about Trump, she says no. We speak by Skype and, for much of our conversation, her two large, sweet-faced dogs are playing in the background, cooped up inside by Virginia's biting January cold snap. Though I can't see the winter out her window, I know exactly what it looks like: the rust-colored ground hardened and shining with frost. It's the winter of my childhood. Prior and I have never met, but, when we talk, I feel an instant kind of familiarity born of a common geography and shared intellectual interests. Prior is both sharp and warm. Like me, she talks with her hands.

As a scholar, Prior specializes in the eighteenth-century British novel, but she's used to being asked to speak on the record about Evangelicalism in contemporary America. She's a Research Fellow with the Ethics and Religious Liberty Commission of the Southern Baptist Convention, and a Senior Fellow with Liberty's own Center for Apologetics and Cultural Engagement. Her faculty profile on the university's website describes her as being drawn to early British literature in part for its emphasis on *philosophy, ethics, aesthetics, [and] community.*

These issues are all at the forefront for Prior. She's been a vocal critic of Trump from inside the Evangelical faith, writing regularly about politics and culture for *Christianity Today* and a variety of other publications, and posting articles on Facebook that sometimes yield comment threads more than a hundred entries long. She thinks Liberty students' support of Trump mostly indicates that he was the one of two bad options they could bear to vote for. Students voted, she said, because, as an institution, Liberty makes the importance of voter turnout clear, and they view it as a responsibility, but in general she sees them as disenchanted with American politics. After the election, they largely seemed neither vindicated nor troubled, eager to move on and to live out their faith in ways they see as more immediate and effective.

Though Prior says she is *mad at everyone* who got us to the point where we were choosing between Trump and Clinton, she has a lot of sympathy for Evangelicals who voted for the president, people like her own parents. She reasons that they feel like Trump's behavior is bad but that, really, *everything is corrupt and base and crass*, and by *everything* she means the whole of the culture around us. She tells me that she and her father love watching *Modern Family* together in the evenings, but that they often cringe at much of the show's overt depiction of sexual behavior. Recalling it, she shudders visibly. I brace, readying for her to draw particular attention to the fact that one of the show's central marriages is between two men, but instead she points out the relationship between the family patriarch and his second wife: a very beautiful, much younger woman who wears high heels and a lot of lipstick. I want to push her here. Isn't voting for Trump just making the debasement of American culture worse? It is, and Prior knows it. But it hits me all at once that *I* feel like *Modern Family* is a truly wholesome show: Every episode I've seen centers on some theme of family togetherness, the importance of hard work, the reasons why it's important to be honest with your partner. It's sweet, goofy, and warm. I try to imagine feeling so outside of what I see as *American culture* that I find this show, even in moments, offensive and crass. I can't. This whole discussion seems like rationalizing an unconscionable choice to me. But Prior seems to think many Evangelicals, especially older ones, feel mainstream culture as a kind of onslaught, that there are faithful Evangelicals who voted for Trump, utterly wearied by the culture around them, thinking: *At least he's a successful businessman,* or *Lord, there's no way he can make anything worse.*

Prior is a contributor to the new anthology *Still Evangelical? Insiders Reconsider Political, Social, and Theological Meaning.* In her essay, she identifies the presence and cultivation of an individual social conscience as one of the hallmarks of Evangelicalism. Yet she sees Liberty students as largely uninterested in politics as a primary ground on which to express this social conscience, or live out their faith. I press her on why; it has to be more than just the absence of an ideal candidate. In response, she pauses and tilts her head slightly up toward the ceiling, a tic I'm learning means she's searching not just for the right language in which to express herself, but for the exact nature of her thoughts. First, she makes an argument I've heard others make about political engagement and millennials: essentially, that it isn't immediate enough. Today's Liberty students, she points out, were raised in the age of social media, and they're used to their interactions with celebrities, or people in power, being instantaneous and informal, modulated by Facebook or Instagram. They post a comment, someone replies. Prior tells me that, just recently, she was reading a letter to the editor in her local paper in which someone was lamenting having to fill out an official form on Virginia congressman Bob Goodlatte's website, provide their contact information, and wait for an aide to be in touch. For the letter writer, she says, the act felt *hard and distant*—too formal, too slow. They wanted a more immediate way to be in touch with people in power.

It's only after we discuss the ways that social media seems at odds with the pace of formative political and cultural change that Prior alights on a second, more intriguing theory. *Evangelicals are famous*, she says, laughing, f*or commonly asking one another: Can you name the day and the hour you were saved?* According to the doctrine Prior believes in, salvation is instantaneous and immediate. Evangelicalism is a faith that de-emphasizes spiritual formation, and even good works, in favor of a single moment in which you accept the Lord as your savior and are brought into the family of God. Once you're saved, you can't be unsaved, and you're brought into heaven by *faith alone.*

For Evangelical believers, the most important decision in one's life—in some ways, the only choice that really matters—occurs abruptly, in the direct presence of God and other people, and then can't be undone. Salvation is necessarily instantaneous and immutable, fundamentally unlike the glacial back and forth of politics, the way power changes hands and people change sides, all of it somehow both infuriatingly slow and unfathomably small in contrast to the Kingdom of God.

These thoughts are new for Prior; she acknowledges that she's never before tried to verbalize them in relationship to politics. In talking, we arrive at her sense that many of today's Liberty students feel doubly removed from politics, alienated both generationally and by virtue of the timing and scale of their faith. Her students, she says, still remain deeply committed to the Evangelical ideals of witness and commitment to social service and change, but they want to enact that change on a one-to-one basis: in ministry, through business, through the arts, in person-to-person conversations in bookstores. They want to see the Kingdom of God spread from individual to individual, watching the instant of salvation light like a candle flame in one life, then another. Another life changed, and another soul saved, no matter who is sitting in the Oval Office.

When I ask her how she copes with being part of a faith tradition she feels is riddled today with so many *foibles* (her word) or being publicly associated with a university that has a presence on America's stage as a bastion of Trump and his politics, Prior talks about reminding herself daily of both the fundamental truths she believes in and of how much better things are now than they were a few hundred years ago, *when church leaders and government leaders could burn . . . torture, enslave people at will.* On the one hand this feels like a flimsy and convenient rationalization: *Even if Trump's behavior is awful, at least we're not burning people alive anymore.* But on the other hand, I understand on some emotional level what she means: I've always liked how the Church makes me feel small, my own body and life dwarfed by God's scale, and by the fabric of the long history of the Church unfurled before me. I resist the urge to point out to Prior that this is what I love most about being Catholic, the sense that it ties me to a tradition that goes back, and back, and back to something sturdy. Multiple times, Prior uses the same metaphor: *Once you're born, you can't change your birth parents.* In other words, once you're part of the Family of God, there's no getting lost, getting abandoned, or getting out. *I'm comfortable with conflict, and with tensions,* she says. She knows that no matter what tradition she was practicing, she'd feel those and acknowledge them. She believes what she believes, and she's certain about it. This is a steadying force. I wonder if it's also a limiting one.

*

When I go home to visit my parents in Virginia over the holidays, I never go to church because my parents don't. Asking them to take me feels like an imposition, though I know they'd agree in an instant. Instead, my father and I sit on the couch with our laptops and trade recommendations of new music we've discovered in the past several months, or my mother and I have lunch at a nearby winery and discuss the classes she'll teach in the upcoming semester. Outside the tasting room's tall glass windows, the Blue Ridge Mountains are purple in the distance, a whole slate of uninterrupted sky above and around them. Looking at that vista, I always think, *Something made this*. It's a view that makes me believe in God in that instinctual way I have no language for. Like a reflex. Like the way my heart beats. Driving by Liberty's campus, with its brick buildings, one after the other, expressionless and vast, I feel the opposite: vacant and hollow. All I think is, *I don't like what's here.*

But, for Prior, God is profoundly present on those grounds. She feels free to do her job at Liberty in a way she knows she wouldn't at a secular university. She can teach whatever texts she likes, from *Jane Eyre* to *Fun Home*, and, to hear her describe it, the university always has her back in the event that a parent complains about her reading list. (She doesn't feel like Liberty's day-to-day operations are influenced by Falwell Jr.'s politics, except maybe when it comes to who speaks at the school's regular convocation.) But Prior believes there's a divine and scriptural truth at the bottom of everything her students study, everything about the world. And the fact that her students share this foundation, and the university supports it, makes all the difference. She's taught at secular schools before, where she describes feeling alienated and judged for the nature and extent of her faith. But it's more than that. The difference, she says, between discussing a text while centering the biblical and spiritual foundation of the issues it addresses, and analyzing it without a shared spiritual focus, is like the difference between looking at a dead moth, pinned to a cork board, and a live one, beating its wings and breathing in the light. Her students, she explained, trust her explicitly because they know she shares their faith, and she can push them to interrogate their assumptions and even their politics (or lack thereof) in a way they wouldn't tolerate if they didn't share that common Evangelical foundation.

Prior rarely prays with her students in class, but she describes one seminar group being so collectively moved by the Cynthia Ozick story "The Shawl" that, instead of formally closing class when the bell rang, she just quietly asked them to pray together. I imagine them in one of Liberty's huge brick classroom buildings. Several students cried, she tells me. She nearly tears up recounting it. *That was, like, the most powerful moment in all my years of teaching,* she says, adding that she thinks it couldn't have happened like that anywhere else. I have to admit she's probably right.

Here's what happens in "The Shawl:" A woman on a forced march to a Nazi concentration camp, cold as the "coldness of hell," conceals her baby in a shawl that, even as she herself starves, sustains the infant. The baby sucks the fabric as her mother's milk dries up and, miraculously, survives. Eventually, though, an older child—desperate, and jealous, and cold—snatches the shawl away, and the baby begins to howl. When a guard discovers the baby, he picks her up and throws her into an electric fence, where she hangs *like a butterfly touching a silver vine.* Voices in the air tell the mother to run to her child, but instead she stands rooted, sucking on the recovered shawl. She knows that if she moves, she'll die.

When I imagine Prior and her students moved to silence, then to prayer, bent over Ozick's story, two things strike me at once. The first is that, though Ozick is Jewish, the story is one about the very kind of mystical salvation Evangelicals believe in. In the darkest moment, in a place like hell, a baby is sustained by something as simple as a shawl imbued with an inexplicable power much bigger than its materiality. The second is that it's also a story about how people—mortal, fallen, and flawed—ruin that salvation in horrifying ways, with their need, their selfishness, and a hatred so large and violent it turns infants into insects, electrocuted in barbed wire.

When I look at Trump, I see hatred just as big, obvious, and destructive. His politics are costing people their dignity and their lives, and his hatred threatens to dwarf whatever shawl of faith I wrap myself in. Certainty is dangerous if it allows you to turn your head away from such destruction, to endorse it even passively. And yet it's true that I often bow my head in prayer when moved by stories or by suffering. It's true that I want nothing more than to be sure that God will answer.

PUBLIC ANATOMY

We return to some spaces in the world because we enter them and feel that they were made for us. Others, we come back to because we wish that they were. And still others pull us back despite our resistance, despite the grief they cause us, like there's some filament—fine and strong as fishing line—stretched from a hook in our cheek all the way to that ground. For me, the anatomical theater in Bologna's first medical school is each of these spaces at once. This is the room where the earliest formal human anatomy classes were conducted, where doctors did some of the first scientific dissections of human bodies in the West. I'm here sixteen months to the day after the first time I ever saw it. I am looking again at the marble dissection table; at the two skinless men, whittled from wood to sinew up on the wall; at the figures representing fourteen constellations carved into the ceiling, bodies which look now, in a way I don't remember from before, like they are caught in a perpetual fall.

*

The rest of the city is profoundly unfamiliar: the streets, the language, the customs, and the light. I'm here alone, on a writing fellowship with no built-in structure, and I often go whole days without speaking to anyone, rolling my wheelchair along Bologna's smoothest porticos and turning left or right wherever there's a sudden set of stairs or the tile gives way to unnavigable cobblestones, letting my body's limits and the city's architecture dictate my path. I eat very little, both because the combined barriers of language and the high stone ledges into most of the cafes and restaurants frequently feel incapacitating, and because my appetite has all but evaporated. Instead, I make slow wheeling circles through the city's center until I find a place with outdoor tables where I can order an espresso or a drink and graze on the peanuts or chalky Italian crackers that come along with it. Or I sit and pick at small bowls of pasta at street-side tables. I read novels until the sun starts to set, or scan the news from the States, which is never good. In the dark, I go back to the apartment that I'm renting; keep my eyes on the street, watching for abrupt changes in terrain. This becomes routine astonishingly quickly, the whole world narrowed to a little maze. It's only as it gets colder and the sun starts setting earlier and earlier, that I zip my jacket up to my chin, shivering at a metal cafe table, and realize soon it will be a problem that I've found almost nowhere where I can get inside alone to eat a meal.

*

Every space in the city has had so many lives. A few blocks from my apartment there's a shell-pink group of buildings that are now part of a university, but which, in the centuries and centuries they've stood, have been municipal offices, a monastery, a funerary space, and a prison. Now there are books lofted in the high, barred windows that used to belong to jail cells, and undergrads in inexplicable silk-screened t-shirts (which read things like *Go Go Go!* above a picture of a frog) studying where monks once prayed and bodies once lay, waiting for burial. The whole city is this spectacular kind of palimpsest—all its past selves visible under the transparent film of its present—and so is also a doubled memento mori. Every building is lit up with centuries of proof that it will outlast us all, and also—with its narrow halls and doors, its windy stairs and lofted rooms—with the reminder that it comes from a time when a body like mine would never have survived, an era when my whole life would have been just an instant of impossibility. And so every day that I wake up here, I go out into these great dueling benedictions and admonitions: Be grateful, you are small and brief and breathing. Be careful, you are small and brief and breathing.

*

I keep a mental catalog of all the buildings it looks like I could enter without pain or trouble: shop selling cheap plastic cellphone cases covered in fish, rhinestones, and flowers; men's tailor; what must be a pawn shop, with a strange constellation of old boom boxes, jewelry, and sports equipment in the front widow; a bridal boutique. Quickly, I learn that my best bet is major chains: McDonald's, the Apple Store, the perpetual neon of the H&M. It's strange to see these corporations transplanted into this ancient city, taking over milky marble rooms with industrial fryers and faux leather leggings, but it's even stranger to reckon with the ways they make me realize capitalism is really the only force that's carved any kind of place for my body in this extraordinary city—some corporate policy that reads in summary, *We build ramps in all our stores so that, no matter what, you can come in and spend your money*. Most of the churches in the city don't have obvious ramps unless they're also tourist attractions, but the automatic doors of the boutique Best Western have been retrofitted so that they're exactly flush with the street. I understand these corporations' motives; I'm frequently disgusted by their politics; I would resent their intrusion into any landscape I loved. They're the part of the city I want least, charmless places, vacated of layered meaning. But when I discover that the Apple Store has a bathroom with elevator access, big enough that I can use it in the wheelchair, I cry a little at the sink before I leave it. I've been limiting the amount of water I allow myself to drink during the day because I'm afraid of ending up desperate to pee with nowhere to go.

*

The first time I watch a woman cross herself in the street when I approach, I think I must have misconstrued the situation, missed some unfamiliar cultural cue. I move past her and try to forget it. But the second time, the old man looks right at me as he makes the gesture, shuffles back away from me into the street, his face so devastated that I have a brief, fierce urge to comfort him. But then he turns away, and I'm left enraged. At first I'm sure that he's mourning something ruined in the combination of my youth, my disability, and my femininity: some wrecked potential for beauty, vitality, fertility, whatever. Then, I think that he's warding off whatever horrible accident he assumes befell me, like I'm a vampire spreading the contagion of misfortune. Hardly sleeping, ill at ease, and entirely solitary, I do feel—to be honest—a little vampiric.

Only later do I wonder whether he caught me staring up and through the doors along the street that we were moving down: the perfumery, the little bookstore hung with ornate maps, the bakery, the narrow shop with a gray dress in the window so beautiful I just wanted to hold it. I had been peering into every one wishing that I could go inside, trying not to pause too long at any single place. I wonder if what actually moved him to the gesture was the largeness and clarity of my desire, the transparency of my grief.

*

I have spent the last month almost swallowed by the force of my desire, not just for entrance into the many pieces of this city that deny me access, but for another body entirely. I blame the one I have for the obvious things: the places I can't go; the amount of pain I'm in; the fact that I don't have the energy or the wherewithal to start Italian lessons, to figure out how to take the bus out to the modern art museum or even to stumble through a clumsy conversation with the friendly bartender—the energy to make a life for myself here. But I blame it for other things, too. I blame it for making me feel selfish all the time, because my attention is turned so thoroughly inward, attending to its needs. I blame it for my fear that my writing will always be narrow, hemmed in by its hurt and relentlessness. I blame it for screwing with my plans, for always demanding revision to fit its stringent reality. I blame it for the fact that I'm alone here, though I chose it. I watch a young mother in a yellow scarf muscle her baby in a stroller up a sidewalk curb, and I blame my body. I watch a man leap up to restrain his old dog as a bicycle passes, and I blame my body. I watch a woman hold a door open with her hip while she sips a coffee, and I blame my body: for all these flashes of lives that will never be mine.

Above all, though, I blame my body for the fact that, after all these years, I'm still grieving a plain stupid grief that I can't hide. I blame it for being itself, for existing to be ruined and repaired.

*

The anatomical theater is not a cathedral. But like a church, it is a place where men once pushed against the contours of the known, past what was immediately visible, toward something more magnificent, mysterious, and powerful. It is a place where they asked, *What makes us who we are?* Now it's a museum of the things we know and don't know about the body. A fraught and complicated monument to how we learned them, what we call error, and how we reach in to alter, inscribe, and repair it. To what's gained—and lost—in the remaking, and all the violence and tenderness done in the name of that project, today and for centuries before. It's the place a man first learned the things that would save and shape me. That would let me walk. That would fail to let me walk well. That would yield both my range of motion and my scars. That would mean I could travel to this country alone. That I could enter a pawn shop, but not so many ancient churches. It's here they began to make a knowable place of my body by naming its parts. This room is the reason I don't remember myself before a man opened me up and altered my wiring. My first memory is a surgical theater. This is as close to the beginning as I can go, just to learn that I can't stay.

A Brief Litany Of Forgettings

Just beyond the apartment building where I'm staying in London, there are train tracks running by the river. The stretch below my window is busy all day with railroad cars peeling continually by. But, somehow, I only ever hear the train at night. And when it wakes me from sleep, sounding so much more like a sudden rush of water than any machine, I am not in England, or nearly thirty, or tangled in the rough, unfamiliar duvet my landlady left on an unfamiliar bed. For a brief stretch of seconds, I am always in Virginia, in the little sleigh bed that was my mother's before it was mine, and it's always winter, and the train outside is the freight train of my childhood, cutting sideways through a blue hill, carrying coal.

It's one of the most magical features of memory: the way a version of the world attaches to the noise of a distant train and then hangs on through decades, with enough brute strength to momentarily unseat the whole, real present when the train churns past you in another life. How the shadow of a prior continent eclipses so completely where you are. How thoroughly you can forget your current self.

*

We tend, I think, to think of forgetting as a failure of memory: *I forget her name. I forgot we saw her.* Or, as some failure of our past self to act: *I forgot to call you back. I forgot I said I'd go.* The word has no true synonyms in English, and every approximation suggests error: *neglect, omit, abandon, overlook, fail to think of, fail to recall.* These approximations cast forgetting as a lack of energy, the absence of attention or activity. Forgetting as foundering, erasure, a match going out.

In my own life, forgetting often feels yoked so closely to grief that they're nearly inseparable. Forgetting as loss: the years of my childhood when I could walk a city block, or head off down to the beach alone, consigned now to the realm of invention and make-believe. The body that chased my brother, stumblingly, through the fields behind the house where we were raised, replaced by the present version of my shape, the current limits of my motion, my current pain. When the train churning outside returns me, for a moment, to my past, the body it evokes is always, only, still. The version of my childself who moves forgotten irrevocably.

And then, there is the kind of loss too total even for forgetting: the stretches of time when I was under anesthesia washed falsely blank in chemicals. The body I was born with, the one that existed un-breached, before anyone had ever cut me open. The months before memory was viable, when I was a twin in the womb, when she had a heartbeat, and I could hear it, and her body was still becoming itself. When her future self had not yet failed to breathe. When we were just accumulation. When we were.

Forgetting as impossible. The utter absence of memory a punishment for living on without her.

This litany is old, and so familiar I know it like a prayer. My intimate and potent catalog of what I don't have anymore, of what I have forgotten, of what didn't last long enough even to forget. The other day I wrote to someone, *I am made up of forgetting,* and then thought better of the melodrama of the line. The specifics of my blankness—stretched through and beyond forgetting—are mine alone, but everyone is marked by gaps in memory, stretches of dark, the way the pieces of life recede into the distance until you lose them over the horizon behind you.

It's a feature of being alive: forgetting as inevitable, as slippage, as a consequence of time.

But last night, I woke again to the passing train. And in that bleary, blue-lit window just beyond being asleep, I forgot again for a moment where or who I was, and forgetting didn't feel like absence, slippage, or loss, but like the tautening of some central muscle: powerful and total. And I've been thinking, again, about what it means to be made of forgetting, not just as an accumulation of losses, failures, absences and caverns, but as a kind of constitutive force. Forgetting as a means of survival.

*

There's a distinction to be made here, between forgetting and ignoring. When you ignore something, you see it, still, in the corner of your vison. You know it's there, you just refuse to fully turn your head. This is a tactic I take all the time with daily chronic pain: feel it, but decline to attend. It's one I use if I decide to try to climb a flight of stairs, or stand up in the classroom or at a party. I know the consequence is out there waiting, and I choose to pretend otherwise, to deal with the aftermath when it arrives. Ignoring comes in handy with the constant stares of strangers. I know they're looking, but I will not look for them. It's a mostly benign tool, with obvious, immutable limits. A blunt blade.

Forgetting is another creature. When you forget something, it really does evaporate, traceless and gone. You can train yourself into it with practice, endurance, and commitment. But it's a sharp and complicated tool.

The dangerous kind of forgetting begins at the limits of ignoring's refusal, at the place where years of declining to look at your standing body in the mirror, to attend to the truth of your own motion, to imagine in any real detail future versions of your life which include a wheelchair, your increasing inability to climb a flight of stairs, or the fact that you will never teach a class standing up or hold a child on your hip, yields to the erasure of those truths in your own imagination, the erasure of the parts of yourself that are shaped by those realities. Your hold on who you really are begins to disappear, and you're left instead with a version of yourself who is half shadow and chasm, who disintegrates to nothing when you try to comprehend the whole of her.

If you leave unattended the blankness this kind of forgetting creates, it will undo you and leave nothing in its wake. But an emptiness doesn't have to be a wound. Forgetting has potential energy, another face.

*

Even as a child, I was a ravenous memorizer of poems. Some of this was because my parents are writers who thrilled at my attention to books, and I never got tired of their palpable delight when I recited the opening lines of poems: Auden's *As I walked out one evening,* or Hopkins' *Glory be to God for dappled things*; Dickinson's *I felt a funeral in my brain,* or Shakespeare's *Let me not to the marriage of true minds /admit impediments.* But even more than their obvious joy, I loved the strange immersive music, loved being able to call up these small, whole worlds on command. I used to put myself to sleep that way, speaking them out loud, into the dark: Donne's *Batter my heart, three-person'd God;* Roethke's *The whiskey on your breath / could make a small boy dizzy;* Dickinson, again: *I am afraid to own a body* . . .

For a long time, I wouldn't have said this had anything at all to do with forgetting. If anything, I would have located in it only the opposite, the pleasure of recollection. This, I would have said, is how a writer gets trained—how she learns attention, and rhythm, structure, repetition, and image, and line. And that's all true, but it's only a piece of it. There's a reason I needed the poems to sleep, a reason I needed to vocalize another world. If I could get the whole thing right—*this Mortal Abolition*—make the music present and exact, then I could replace myself with it entirely, and I could make that substitution last. I could forget myself completely for as long as I could conjure up *the Shreve High Football Stadium* or *sawdust restaurants with oyster shells* and hold them, real there in the air. And I would have no body, bucking madly against plaster casts; no braces propped like some limbs, badly salvaged, in the corner of my room; no strange and incurable loneliness I couldn't account for except as my sister's shape. The erasure was utter. I was bodiless, gone entirely except as voice and listener, composed solely of someone else's language. Just metaphor. Just music.

This was a useful kind of forgetting. I learned to do it when I was frequently desperate to be gone, when I might instead have hurt myself, tried more damaging tactics to engender my own disappearance. It's still my favorite part of really entering a poem, how it overrides me with its own body, swallows me to nothingness. Natasha Trethewey writes, *I make between my slumber and my waking. / It's as if you slipped through some rift, a hollow. / I was asleep while you were dying*, and I slip away into the world of her language.

I make between my slumber and my waking. / It's as if you slipped through some rift, a hollow. / I was asleep while you were dying. Trethewey's lines, remembered and repeated, have enough weight to dislodge the loud, savage fact of my body. Like the train that passes underneath my bedroom window, they replace its truth with another one. And the version of the world they make appear has, not the ephemeral shimmer of some half-asleep recollection, but substance and staying power. A poem belongs not just to dreaming, but to the waking world.

*

If the space forgetting engenders is an emptiness, a missing thing, a wound, then it is also the field burned on purpose, without panic, to make it fertile for another crop. It's also the blank page, the clear expanse that waits for Donne's *little world made cunningly / of elements and angelic sprite.* It's a station where the train halts, briefly, before continuing on.

*

Not the end of the line, but a pausing place. The quiet that begets invention, makes the next thing reachable, possible, real.

Fragments, Never Sent

D*ear F,*

Throughout high school and college, when I was trying to be a writer, I also tried, regularly, to be a person who kept notebooks, because I understood it is what writers do: Joan Didion at the *hotel bar, Wilmington RR* on an *August Monday morning.* Our father, always with a black Moleskine and a bleeding Pilot pen. I knew I was supposed to be paying attention, taking notes, feeling my head fill up with fragments of language I couldn't afford to forget. So I bought journals, and began them, and left them off, and bought others, and did it again. It's not surprising I was never any good at it: It's hard for me to write more than a few sentences by hand before my spastic fingers start to hurt, and then my wrist, and then my arm if I press on for long enough. And, anyway, I'm too precious about objects, too opposed to error, for that kind of record keeping: the whole book always seemed ruined once one page was ugly, or false-started, or banal. But that's less than half the story. I still have all those partial notebooks, boxed up in a storage unit with the rest of what I own, because I am a writer now, and working on a project somewhere between permanent addresses. And, though I haven't really looked at them in years, I know that nearly every started page is fashioned not just as a note, or fragment, or idea, but as a letter meant for you. They all begin *Dear Frances, Dear Franny, Dear F, Dear Sister, Dear Ghost.*

Then, mostly, I go on to talk about the weather, or the book I'm reading, something I overheard, someone I'm drawn to: as if you know what *summer* is, or *September,* or *coffee* or the *radio* or *Jupiter* or a *bruise* or the *stretch of Highway 1 that runs up California's coast.* As if you've ever seen a *cliff.* Everything is something I want to tell you. Or, the whole world feels remarkable when I imagine you in it. Or, often when I'm bored, or crabby, I remember you are dead and have never run your fingers through your hair, or lit a match, or looked out of a car window or heard anybody call for you across a room, and that knowledge makes things sharp and worthwhile again.

But, after a few paragraphs of any letter, I always run into the fact that I don't know you at all. That you're just a figure I've made up in relief against myself. An imaginary friend, continually conjured way past childhood. An absence I've spent a lifetime papering around. You're just the page, and anything I write to you is selfish. You're a way to lend more weight to what I'm saying to the air.

*

Dear F,

I've been collecting stories about separated twins since I was old enough to look for them. Castor and Pollux hatch from a single egg and grow up riding white horses of foam formed by the ocean waves. When Castor dies in battle, Pollux asks to be a star positioned alongside him rather than go on living alone. Given the choice, he'd rather keep his brother than his body. In an updated *Parent Trap,* which I watched hundreds and hundreds of times, two versions of Lindsay Lohan discover one another at summer camp. They reunite their parents, do the rest of their growing up together. In a newspaper article, two brothers, adopted to different families at birth, know nothing about one another. They are both named Jim. They both get married twice, first to women named Linda, then to women named Betty. They pick up identical smoking habits; they both have dogs named Toy. They live forty-five miles apart, but don't meet until they're 39. They discuss their identical tension headaches and woodworking hobbies. Move in next door to one another. Are never apart again.

When I was a child, I used to imagine one day I'd discover you were out there somewhere living a parallel life. I wanted your death to be a fiction because then my loneliness would be a fiction. And, *look*, I've done it again, arrived already at the selfishness of missing who you could have been for me.

*

Dear F,

Sometimes I think I want to make a list of the things you did feel, and know, when you were alive, those hours when you were. Right here in the world. *The air. The fabric of a hospital blanket. The skin on more than one set of hands. The small heat another body makes while it holds you.* But the list is only solid and comforting like that for a moment before it includes: *The heart monitor yowling. A tube down your tiny throat. Pressure. Electrodes peeling off your skin. Pain. The burning when you can't breathe.* I've had so many tubes down my throat, when I was old enough to recall them. I want none of that for you. I wrote, once, that I wanted a body for you, and it's true. But this is what our body means, as much as any of the rest of it. I should say *bodies.* But now there's only mine and the way it holds the ghost of yours.

*

Dear F,

This is my second year of living, essentially, out of a suitcase. Two Julys ago I paid two men and their wives to pack up the apartment where I'd lived through graduate school and move everything I own into an improbably small storage unit off a highway on the outskirts of a town in Mississippi: All my books, my framed artwork; my bed and the bulk of my cloth-ing; the huge, cheap corkboard where, for years, I'd pinned drafts of poems in progress and postcards from people I loved. I left my guitar there; the black cowboy boots I'd bought and had refurbished when I lived in Texas; the two stuffed sheep that belonged to the two of us in the NICU, wrapped in a blanket, safely in their own box. They're the only thing I own that you ever touched.

I spent a few weeks visiting our parents in Virginia, and then ten months in Arkansas for a short-term job at a literary magazine. Before I arrived, the magazine's staff outfitted an apartment for me, furnished with donations, garage sale finds, and the labor of volunteers. Because they were kind and conscientious, and because they knew the move was jarring and disorienting in the way such temporary relocations often are, they devoted a lot of attention to ensuring the apartment didn't feel sterile and staged. They hung framed paintings on the walls, left a woven throw-blanket on the couch and a blue clay rooster with wire legs on the little kitchen table. The whole place was haphazard and warm, but without any of my own things, it had the effect of making me feel, in the months I lived there, as if I'd stepped into the frame of someone else's life, someone with their own particular taste, and rhythms, and eccentricities. On the phone with friends, I joked wryly that I sometimes had the sensation I'd ousted the apartment's previous inhabitant and just assumed her life in the middle of a workweek; sat down on her beat-up green couch, used her checkered oven mitts, her scuffed blender, her blue poly-blend towels as if they belonged to me, as if no one would notice I had taken her place.

What I didn't tell anyone: Occasionally, I convinced myself the room around me was filled not with the cast-offs of strangers, but with things you had accumulated and loved. That it was your life I'd stepped suddenly into the center of: quotidian, tangible, ongoing. I picked up the soap dish in the bathroom: a cheap plastic clamshell, just some beachfront souvenir, and felt a rush of tenderness, thought, *Thank God, she's been to the ocean.*

*

Dear F,

I always think of you more around our birthday, but the summer I turned twenty, I couldn't stop thinking, *She'll have been dead for twenty years.* Something about the roundness of the number, the magnitude of two decades, some presumed arrival of my own adulthood, threw your absence into sharp relief. I dreamed about you every night for weeks. You were always far away, across a river or a wide field, looking back at me with my own eyes. You were always still and sitting on the ground. You never came for me, or reached toward me, but you looked and looked. In the dreams, I always had to be the one to walk away and leave you.

*

Dear F,

You come to me at the strangest times. It isn't always my face that does it, although that's an easy trigger. More often, actually, it happens when I am putting on my shoes and my eye catches on the slight, pale plank of my foot, or when I am calling to someone across a great distance and I hear my own voice ringing in the air. A man brings my hand slowly to his mouth, kisses the heel of my palm. My first thought: *This could be your hand.* And then: *You'll never have a lover.*

*

Dear F,

I wonder how often our mother looks at me and misses you.

*

Dear F,

We were born too early to have ever opened our eyes. I just realized that means we never saw each other.

*

Dear F,

I hope you weren't afraid.

FRANKENSTEIN ABROAD

The winter of my freshman year of college I broke into a house. It was alone on a hill that bordered the rural New England campus, and I'd passed by it almost every day for months on a route my friend M and I looped in the evenings, when we were sick of our reading and needed air. Those months, we talked a lot about being young and smart and unhappy. We traded music recommendations, and I mulled over going to Divinity School, which I knew nothing about, but liked the sound of. She hummed bars of the songs she was writing and recounted her linguistics lectures, and we smoked the occasional cigarette, which seemed, then, like something you had to do if you were going to live in the middle-of-nowhere Massachusetts, and talk about *Hamlet* all the time, and never sleep. In my memory, this is how we spent most of that year.

We were barely seventeen, and that winter everything we saw seemed beautiful because it was difficult: the spare, gold plant that grew along the road even in the snow; each other's cheekbones; the stray, dark bodies of the last geese in the fields. Even the lake, frozen a turbid gray that made me want to head out onto the water just to test the strength of the ice. It was cold all the time, so we wore scarves and fur-lined boots and coats with high collars, and we blew on our hands.

The house was where we always stopped and turned around, pausing at the crest of the hill to look down at the scrub grass and the bare branches and all the feet between us and the valley. It was in that shadow state between use and abandonment, and we debated for weeks whether or not it belonged to anyone, drawing steadily closer, peering in the windows and over the low fence at all the ivy growing untamed in the garden. We never saw a car in the driveway, and though I sometimes thought I noted changes in the debris on the front lawn, there were never any certain signs of life.

I don't remember why we finally tested the gate and went inside, only that M found an unlatched window she could clamber through, and then went around and unlocked the front door so I could come inside. The first floor of the house was one large, open room, empty except for some scattered cardboard boxes, an overturned paint can in the fireplace, and a big piano in the middle of the space. M went straight to it and began to play, first softly, and then so loudly I was sure someone would hear and call the police. I wouldn't have dreamed of telling her to be quiet. She sang, and I went through what was left in the kitchen: an unplugged phone, a flashlight without batteries, one of those little yellow note-pads for taking messages, a half a pack of coffee filters, a bright red colander spotted with rust.

I was a sucker for the intense specificity of what had been abandoned, for the way the piano in the background suggested a soundtrack, for the sense that this could be a scene from every movie I had ever loved. We found partly full boxes, and, in my head, a voiceover played: *Through a window you see two girls, seated on the floor, stripping off their coats and shoes and sweaters piece by piece. The light is copper and thick around them, and they pull things slowly from the boxes. You can see a quilt, a gilded picture frame, two candle-sticks, a lighter. One of them looks down at a photograph and puts her thumb to a face on the glass. The other tucks her hair behind one ear. They don't speak. You want, madly, to be close to them, and whatever it is they are discovering there.*

To be just a little wild and subversive in a way that was magnetic rather than repellant. To take the stupid, minor risks of youth because I felt a sturdiness I could trust at the bottom of my own life. To be lovely, even just in freeze-frame, in a house that wasn't mine, my loneliness the compelling and resolvable kind. That was everything I wanted.

That same winter, I read *Frankenstein* for the first time.

It was part of a class titled Milton and Aftertimes, a sur-vey of the poet's major works followed by contemporary texts that owed them some debt. I had a brilliant young professor, and I loved the course from the outset. We read *Lycidas* and *Samson Agonistes,* and then I memorized the opening stanzas of *Paradise Lost: of Man's First Disobedience, and the Fruit / Of that Forbidden Tree, whose mortal taste / Brought Death into the World, and all our woe.* I felt personally offended when we reached *Paradise Regained* and it was bad in comparison, all the complication of an exiled Satan, *Paradise Lost's* superior inventor, flattened by the dogma of an eternally smug and victorious Jesus.

And then we came to *Frankenstein.*

The story at the center goes like this: Victor Frankenstein, a young and brilliant man raised in Italy, has a life marked by privilege, then grief. His mother dies of scarlet fever, and he goes to university occupied with the *deepest mysteries of creation,* intent on learning how to make a living being so that he might combat loss, death, and decay. He does it, sutures a man from salvaged parts he selects because they're perfect in proportion, then animates the body that he's made. But the Creature, wonderful as it is in theory, horrifies him once it breathes, and starts, and wants him. He abandons the miserable monster he made, and the Creature, in its wretched loneliness, begs, *Don't disdain me.* Then, when it is still abhorred, ruins its creator's life, the lives of the people he loves. It's a story of almost no consolation. One that ends in darkness and ice, the Creature on the ocean floating away from the dead body of the man who made him, in misery and mourning.

The first time the Creature moves, wakes into the world on the table where it has been stitched together, *a convulsive motion agitate[s] its limbs,* and the sight of that spasm is enough to let Frankenstein know he's made a grave and irredeemable error. I've woken up in spasm every morning of my life, and, the first time I read that description, I felt my own legs contract in recognition. But the thing that struck me most acutely, then, was the novel's certainty, right from the outset, that a being who is perfect in pieces and proportion, flawless in its stilled fragments, can, when it is sutured and set back in motion, become a *wretch* and a *catastrophe,* an object of abject horror. The book knows the way a body becomes most monstrous when it wakes and tries to walk.

At seventeen, I was obsessed with the origins of the way I moved: with how I came into the world thirteen weeks early, weighing just over two pounds; with how many minutes of oxygen deprivation it took to cause the brain damage that left me disabled; how many minutes made the difference between my life and my twin sister's death; with how surgeons had split and sewn me on a table, remade me, watched me wake, watched a *convulsive motion agitate [my] limbs,* evidence of an irreparable error in my composition; with the question of whether, somewhere inside themselves, they felt something like horror stir.

I was only a year out of full-length leg braces that extended from my hip to my ankle. They had metal hinges that locked and unlocked when I pulled a big, rubber-coated handle behind my knee, and when I stood, they held my legs completely straight. In them, I walked using crutches in front of my body, swinging my legs out from my hips like planks of lumber. I moved remarkably like Boris Karloff playing Frankenstein's monster in the 1931 film: stiff-legged, scarred, and undead. I came to college on the run from that version of myself.

Even at seventeen, I knew enough to feel slightly ridiculous in my identification, to locate something absurd and melodramatic in a tiny blue-eyed girl with spastic legs and a lurching gait professing to see herself in a sallow-skinned giant constructed from corpses. But I still have my first copy of the novel, so I know that when I reached the scene that finds the Creature asking: *Cursed, cursed creator! Why did I live?* I underlined the question twice.

A decade later, I've reread the novel at least once in nearly every place I've lived.

*

I have a lot of practice being quiet: the years I went to Quaker school, where you sat through a weekly silent meeting, two hundred adolescent bodies shifting in their chairs for forty minutes. The time inside an MRI machine when you can't move or speak, as the machine clangs around you, composing a picture. The long stretch in Mass when the whole congregation files up for communion and, while you should be praying, you watch the way the other women take the wafer in their hands, on their tongues. All the accumulated hours when you live alone, and it's you and the radio on in the kitchen, the way the wind buffets the warped door even when it's closed, a neighbor pacing overhead.

But in Italy, it is a different kind of quiet: hours, days, when I don't say more than a fistful of words to another person, ask for a double espresso in broken Italian, say, *I'm sorry, excuse me, sto bene: I'm fine. I'm fine. I'm fine.* In Italy, I feel myself coming unstitched from the world. I can't seem to make myself adjust to the time change, and so I don't fall asleep until the sun is rising. I wake up past two in the afternoon, cotton-mouthed, guilty, and afraid. Often, I spend an hour just sitting in the ground floor apartment I've rented before I can convince myself to leave it, and, when I drag my wheelchair up and over the threshold and out into the sudden, stubborn sunshine, I feel skinless and scorched.

Because motion has always been a struggle, I've never been a person who sets off into the world without a destination. But, in Italy, I find I lose whole days to aimless wandering, circling the same half mile of the city like a stuck bird, going slowly back and forth past the same café four times before I can bring myself to go up to a table and order a drink. Outside Bologna's public library, I watch some teenagers mugging for the camera by the fountain of Neptune, and a young mother playing with her child on the corner of the wide stairs. She blows the baby a kiss in the air, the same gesture in every country. And when the baby blows one back—that perfect, inexplicable reflex for imitation—there's a moment when their mouths are exactly the same shape, and I wonder if the mother catches it, if she's moved to see herself repeated so precisely in her daughter's face.

Ostensibly this is, at least in part, the kind of watching I am here to do. I've deferred a teaching job at a college in Ohio to take a fellowship to live and write abroad. A year of funded time, when my only obligation is to travel, push toward a second book, and get a wider window on the world. In the last ten years, I've lived in five states, built a life in which I get to make things for a living, converted my obsession with my own beginning into a career fashioning one origin story after another: *It began like this.*

Aware of my own propensity for self-involved myopia—and the way my body's pervasive needs, the limits of its motion, feed it—I've done my best, for years, to keep my gaze trained outward on the intricacies of the world around me.

I pay close attention, and I'm up for every new adventure: yes, always, to the city I've never seen, the four-hour conversation with the stranger on the plane. Yes, to packing my bag, to sneaking into that house, to heading for that river, though I can hardly swim. Yes, to seeing what's behind that door. It's among the things I've come to prize most dearly: the way I've fashioned myself self-sufficient, curious, and game.

Here, though, I worry I've flung myself beyond my depth, that I've put myself in an untenable situation I had all the information to anticipate. I've been here before, on a quick trip to visit a friend. This is a cobblestone city built before 1088. There are essentially no laws governing accessibility in the city center. I'm in chronic pain that gets worse under stress: a constant, full-body pressure, like I'm wearing a lead dress. I know only the most rudimentary phrases in Italian, and I have a body that mandates constant articulation: *I can't do that. This is what's wrong. Is there another way inside? I'm fine.*

I've been telling myself for months that my hesitancy to make detailed plans for my time in Italy is because the real shape of the life Bologna will offer me won't come into focus until I've arrived. But part of me knows that it's because living alone in this city is a ludicrous thing for me to be doing, and that, if I attend too closely to the details, this reality will puncture a vision in which, whether or not I want to admit it,

I am walking down Bologna's painted porticos, shouldering a shopping bag as I go up the stairs, and stepping with no problem through the raised door of a museum, a language classroom, a cathedral, a bar.

My body has been mine for far too long for me to have any business with this fantasy. Watching people milling in clusters around the piazza as the sun sinks over the fountain and turns the whole square copper, I hate the clarity with which I feel the pull of the dream, and the presence, after nearly thirty years, of my anger at the distance between it and the reality of my life. The truth ought to be gift enough. After all, I am awake and breathing here. I have made it all this way.

I'm thinking, at that moment, not of Frankenstein's Creature, but of Frankenstein himself, the passage in the novel, early on, when he laments the whole doomed scope of his project: *And how much happier that man who believes his native town to be the world than he who aspires to become greater than his nature will allow.*

I write to friends in the States that I feel alien here: unmoored and estranged, but the truth is, more than anything, I feel like I've woken up in this city some prior version of myself: a girl I thought I'd managed to outrun in all the intervening years. My whiplash is less a result of all that's foreign and far from home, than of a sense of having been flung backwards in the arc of my own life.

I take my copy of *Frankenstein* out of my satchel. Reread those early pages. Take a photograph of the paperback open on the café table. Caption it: *Frankenstein Abroad.*

*

When the Creature asks, *Cursed, cursed creator! Why did I live?* he isn't asking only why Frankenstein brought him to life. He's wondering why he hasn't, when given the opportunity, torn himself limb from limb, *why, in that instant, did I not extinguish the spark of existence you had so wantonly bestowed?*

I know not, he says, but this isn't quite true. And as soon as he asserts it, he goes on: *Despair had not yet taken possession of me; my feelings were those of rage and revenge. I could, with pleasure, have destroyed the cottage and its inhabitants, and have glutted myself on their shrieks and misery.*

I've told every therapist I've ever seen that I've never been actively suicidal. And this is true, in that I've never actively planned to kill myself. Maybe even in that I've never truly wanted to die, although that feels harder to pin down. What it leaves out, though, are the stretches when the whole of my desire to be alive is just a ribbon of rage in my stomach. I told a priest, once, that I worried I only believed in God because I needed an object for my anger, but even that wasn't the whole truth: Sometimes, I worry I believe in God only because the prospect of my rage, unhemmed by the channel faith provides, is too frightening for me to confront.

Frankenstein's Creature learns to read by discovering a copy of *Paradise Lost,* and sees himself reflected in the Satan in its pages. The banished angel Milton conjures knows *The mind is its own place, and in it self / Can make a Heav'n of Hell, a Hell of Heav'n,* but it's the Creature who understands that the place of your mind becomes a universe you carry, one you'll change the lived-in world around you to reflect. He says, *I, like the arch fiend, bore a hell within me, and finding myself unsympathized with, wished to tear up the trees, spread havoc and destruction around me, and then to have sat down and enjoyed the ruin.*

I have been trying not to say that there are whole stretches of my life when I wanted to breathe only as an act of revenge on the forces that had made me, when I woke up so angry I could feel it in my teeth, when the world I wanted to leave in my wake was all wreck and ravage, littered with scattered trees. I have been trying not to tell you that I don't remember a time before fury, that in what the Creature calls the *original era of my being,* I am already seething.

The whole of *Frankenstein* is framed as a letter, recounting a story, recounting a life, and so the book is shot through with the cognizance of how much narration matters, the knowledge that writing is its own act of creation, volatile and crucial. I have the impulse to pause here—like an aside in a letter—and tell you that I know, still, the melodrama of seeing myself repeated in the monstrous creature in a gothic novel. That there's a long tradition of scholarship on disability and monstrosity. And, most urgently, that I have been lucky, and I have been loved.

*

Those early years in college, I got around campus on a big blue tricycle with a white wire basket and an electric motor that growled like an irritated animal. It got noisier when the weather was bad, which it often was. I roped my crutches into the basket with a bungee cord, and lurched from building to building hauling a backpack heavy with books. However slight my body itself might have been, the whole of me was lumbering, large, and loud.

The first time the Creature sees his own reflection in a pool of water, he is revolted and shocked: *At first I started back, unable to believe that it was indeed I who was reflected in the mirror; and when I became fully convinced that I was in reality the monster that I am, I was filled with the bitterest sensations of despondence and mortification.* Every time I thought about the way my body moved through the world, caught sight of myself crouching forward in the hazy reflection of some window glass, I horrified myself.

Looking back at my teenage years, it's my parents who seem bravest. I didn't feel young, then, because you never do when you are. And I wouldn't have admitted to being either furious or fragile, though I was both those things in direct proportion to one another. I transmuted fear and vulnerability to rage so fluidly that I didn't even realize there had been a conversion. I could barely walk and I had very few practical skills, but I was smart and eager for the world. And because my body left me largely unable to make subtler, slower transitions from childhood to adulthood—isolated from my peers, and occupied with surgery, therapy, and pain—I insisted on leaving for college two years early, on a wrenching as unsubtle as my body: seven hundred miles away to a place I could start over on my own.

Letting me go was the right move. I needed to be in a place where I could take pleasure and refuge in my intellect, and I can trace the writer and the teacher I am now back to the education I got during those years, to the work I read from Milton to *Frankenstein* and on. I needed the physical distance, the clear dividing line between what had been before and what would come, but it was an ugly tearing. There were periods when I hardly left my dorm room, felled by a combination of physical pain and profound depression so inextricably linked that now, in memory, I can't distinguish them from one another. My laundry piled up undone. I picked my cuticles, and bit my lips until they bled. These minor, useless damages I inflicted on myself like they might graft over the larger wound. I snapped at anyone who tried to help, and I was cruel to the people who loved me, ashamed of my shape, my suffering and my need.

The piece most painful to recall: my mother's voice on the telephone, the way she paid a man from the local grocery store to come to my dorm with a box of raspberries and yogurt, crackers and sharp cheddar cheese, because I couldn't manage to climb the hill to the dining hall, and I was hardly eating. How, when she called to check on me, I wept and told her: *Just leave me alone,* when the way I was alone was killing her. When she had let me travel all that distance so that I could try to make a life I loved.

In all the intervening years, she's still often ended our phone calls asking: *Are you eating? Do you have enough food?* an echo of old panic in her voice. Sometimes I'm distracted while we talk, and I don't catch myself before my guilt morphs into anger, a reflexive transformation. I snap at her: *Don't ask me that! I'm fine.*

Frankenstein's Creature reached for his maker, begged, *Don't disdain me.* I couldn't stand the way the woman who had made me offered her own hands.

*

Without planning to, I arrive in Italy just in time for the 200th anniversary of *Frankenstein's* publication. The one woman I know in Bologna—who knows that I love the novel, and that I've been trying, inside the fog of my weeks in the city, to write about it—sends me a notice for the conference at a local university in celebration of the bicentennial. It is, miraculously, held in English, and so we go together, late one afternoon, to listen to a talk.

The library where the conference is held is a collection of stone and stucco buildings faded to a kind of pink that suspends them in perpetual sunset. Like everything in the center of Bologna, they're beautiful in a way that makes you feel keenly ephemeral, that magnifies the quickness of your own small life. My friend lifts my wheelchair up over the clay ledge at the edge of the courtyard, and I step up over the threshold, trying not to wince. While we settle on seats at the edge of the room, she tells me what she knows about the building's long history. She's heard it was once a prison and a mortuary, a military fortress and government office. This is why I fell in love with the city the first time I was here: the way it makes a lightbox from so much of Western history. Look at any one building, and so many centuries of life emerge: people suffering and singing, doing paperwork, and going to their graves within the confines of a single, lasting space.

It turns out the first scholar talking that afternoon is mostly discussing not *Frankenstein,* but Mary Shelley's efforts at training herself in translation, and I write down fragments of points about the relationship between composition and transcription, half imagining that I might later work them into an essay about being a writer in a foreign country. Mostly, though, I think about the section in the novel when the Creature watches a family of cottagers through a crack in their rough-hewn wall. How, for hours, he's fascinated by their daily labor and, in seeing their interactions, is struck by *sensations of a peculiar and overpowering nature . . . a mixture of pain and pleasure.* I remember how he retreats to his own shelter, goes to sleep alone on straw. Everything that follows.

I've been tracking the way the planet of pain in my knees and back is expanding every day, and also the frequency with which I find myself returning to that image of the mother and daughter laughing on the library stairs: how I feel first pleasure, then sadness, then, despite myself, anger. That afternoon, when we're outside again in the sunshine, I look up one more time at the ancient library.

I only have one brief life. I can't stay here.

*

I still keep, in my wallet, a copied passage from a memoir by the writer Emily Rapp, about growing up as a poster child for the March of Dimes. I wrote it down by hand, though the act was laborious and strained:

> *I had been fully invested in the lie that I was able-bodied. I had practiced and perfected this fiction, living within it, and according to its dictates, as if it were*

*a moral framework, rather than a complex system
of self-deception: I did not want to be abnormal, or
less than, because of my grievous, irrevocable, physical flaw, so I had to be abnormally fantastic in order
to compensate. The paradox: being extraordinary
was the only way to be ordinary. This worked to
my advantage in many ways. Motivated by the fear
that I would be worthless if I wasn't hugely successful, I worked hard to achieve my goals. But the fear
that fueled my work-ethic had devastating effects on
my self-image. I had convinced myself that if I admitted my limitations. If I failed in any real or imagined
way, it would ruin my life. Who could love a person so
deformed and scarred . . . how could I have pride in an
embodied existence that was such an abomination? I
thought overcoming my disability was the only way
for me to be loved. Yet I was already deeply loved by
many people, I just couldn't manage to love or accept
myself. The problem was mine.*

The paper the paragraph is copied on is soft, and so worn it's
nearly transparent. I've had it since I was fifteen; I almost
never actually take it out anymore. But I think all the time
about how, even then, I knew I'd need that warning again
and again: *You are not able bodied. You can't live as if you are.*

You cannot let the way you hate yourself become the thing that keeps you isolated and estranged.

It's remarkable how, even with that warning tangible and present on my person nearly all the time, I preformed the same flawed, self-sabotaging fiction for so long.

There were those years in Massachusetts when I couldn't admit the winter was unmanageable, that I was still carting the trauma of a childhood where I couldn't trust my own body, or that there were so many basic things I hadn't learned to do, too fully occupied with the project of surviving.

There was the math class I couldn't pass my senior year of college in California because I couldn't admit to anyone that the brain damage that made my muscles spastic and my balance flawed also impaired my ability to process numbers, space, and visual patterns. Because I couldn't stand to be damaged in yet another way, my intellect—the only good piece of me—now marred and monstrous, too. There were the months I spent afterwards lying about it to everyone who loved me, forced to leave my first stint at graduate school because I was still three credits short of my undergraduate degree.

There was the way, years later, I looked into the eyes of a man who touched me tenderly, and with desire, who said he thought he'd like to stick around, and said: *There's something wrong with you,* just to watch his face fall, because I couldn't imagine that he wasn't lying.

I want to pause here, again, and tell you that I know Frankenstein's Creature was made alien by forces he couldn't control, by the people who shrieked at the sight of him, shrank from his touch. That I know, too, the ways for years I made my own loneliness: sought out distance and extremity, excuses to remove myself, called this ambition, achievement, success.

But, until now, I thought I'd learned the lesson that the girl in that abandoned house in New England needed so desperately—that I'd shaken the worst of my damaging fiction and, with it, cast off the bulk of my cruelty, my self-hatred, the sense of my life as some composite of revenge.

Recently, a driver for a ride share service watched me get into his car. He asked me what was wrong with me, then told me—glancing in his rearview mirror—that he felt sorry for me, because my life would always be a little wasted, a little sadder than if I was unbroken or unscarred. I told him that I love the life I have and wouldn't trade it. And I meant it: I write for a living, still obsessed by the same stories. I am *deeply loved by many people.* I have an existence that is wider than I ever dreamed.

But our pain always comes to collect us.

*

The Royal Opera House in London is grand on a scale I've never seen before in a theater: 2,200 seats in red and gold and a high, domed ceiling that arcs up and up. I'm alone in the back row on the orchestra level. And, on the velvet curtain drawn across the stage, there's a skull and spinal column projected, like an illustration from an anatomy textbook rendered so giant it's nearly divine. I'm here to see a new ballet of *Frankenstein.*

I left Italy for London figuring that, however much I'd dreamed about learning Italian, removing the language barrier would make my year abroad some measure easier. And it has helped, although I have a sort of stranded feeling I can't quite name and I'm spinning my wheels on my second book. I'm months overdue on the manuscript, and I'm wondering whether—even all these miles from every place I've ever called home—I have enough distance from my own past to draw anything meaningful together. The notice about this ballet came in an email advertisement, like something fated. I've read that the central set is an anatomical theater, an operating table. That there's a focus on the body, constructed and coming apart.

The moment the action begins, I'm struck by a central strangeness: this story about a body that's extraordinary in a horrifying way, being recounted by these bodies doing things so extraordinary they're magnetic. Every time a dancer leaps, loops an arm around another person's waist or pirouettes, I think, *Oh God,* and am delighted. Then I feel my own body, heavy as lead, in the chair.

The Creature is danced by a figure in a beige, almost transparent leotard covered in obvious stitching crisscrossing his body, thick and gnarled as new scars. When he starts to life on the constructed operating table, Frankenstein is crouching above him, waiting for his heart to beat, and so they spasm the first instant of the Creature's dance together, that first *convulsive motion,* shared rather than singular. Frankenstein's horror is all the more painful to watch because, in that initial instant, he is the perfect mirror of the Creature that he made.

For much of the ballet, the Creature mostly dances on the margins: the estranged mimic of Frankenstein and his family conducting their lives, of his creator fretting over the horror he has wrought. When the Creature takes center stage to do violence—murder Frankenstein's young nephew, best friend and, finally, his wife—the choreography of killing is quick and decisive. It's preceded by longer sequences when his gestures are gentle, when he tries to bow, reach out his hand. He recoils in tandem with the dancers who recoil from him. Through the whole ballet, he *is* frightening, something about his gestures stiff, animal, and *off.*

The ballet departs from the novel at the end: There's a gun on stage, and rather than succumbing, as he does in the text, to exhaustion and hypothermia, Frankenstein shoots himself in full view of his Creature. It's just the two of them. The Creature cradles his maker's body, lays it down, and then gets up, takes center stage. It only takes a second of him claw-ing at the red seams on his leotard before I realize he is pull-ing at his sutures. He is trying to unstitch himself.

I don't realize I am crying until the lights come up.

*

I have come a long way to realize I've been trying to outrun grief. I don't mean this as simply as it sounds; so rarely are our motivations only one thing or the other. I took this fellow-ship because it is a luxury, an honor, a remarkable opportu-nity. It also allowed me the gesture I know best: to tear myself away, to make myself alone.

I would have told you, once, that the impulse for that tearing was born from a fear of being known, and there's a measure of that in it.

I am coming to understand, though, that the thing I've been most hell-bent on avoiding is the scope of my own mourning. The way it resists my knowledge of my luck, my certainty of the value of my own existence, my faith and every prayer I've ever offered up. To grieve feels disloyal to other people with disabilities. It feels selfish, regressive, and weak. I'm ashamed of it.

But I'm more ashamed that I've become a creature more inclined to tear the trees out of the ground—to wrench her own roots up again and again—than to feel the full force of her own life.

Of course, I'm not a monster, not some feral thing a flawed, grief-stricken creator composed, however many mortal men have had their hands inside my body, stitched me up. I'm animal accident, divine design, or dust—or some improbable composite of the three, the way we all are.

In the theater, I do not unstitch myself. I sit still long after the lights come up. I stay where I am.

ACKNOWLEDGMENTS

I'M GRATEFUL to the following publications, in which earlier versions of some these essays first appeared, sometimes under an alternate title: *Image Journal:* "Bent Body, Lamb," *The New York Times:* "Calling Long Distance," *Oxford American:* "The Cost of Certainty," *The Paris Review:* "If You Are Permanently Lost," Pleiades Press, *The Poem's Country: Place and Poetic Practice:* "The Virginia State Colony for Epileptics and Feebleminded," *The Rumpus:* "Something's Wrong With Me," *Virginia Quarterly Review:* "The Broken Country," and *The Yale Review:* "The Skin You're In."

Hasan Altaf, Eliza Borné, Peter Catapano, Maxwell George, Shara Lessley, Mary Kenagy Mitchell, Emily Nemens, Meghan O'Rourke, and Bruce Snider edited individual essays from this collection. Those pieces, and this book as a whole, are orders of magnitude better for their intelligence, attention and care.

Many organizations offered indispensable time and resources to help make this collection possible. Boundless gratitude to the people at the Civitella Ranieri Foundation, United States Artists, the Amy Lowell Poetry Travelling

Scholarship, the Trust of Jeanette Haien Ballard, the University of Mississippi, and the *Kenyon Review,* for their support. Special thanks to the phenomenal folks at the *Oxford American,* who provided me not only with a year to work on this manuscript, but with the kindest, funniest, and most imaginative community I could have asked for.

I'm grateful to the Wellcome Collection in London and the Archiginnasio of Bologna for allowing me into the spaces that inspired many of these essays, to Karen Swallow Prior for our candid and generative conversations, and to Judith E. Heumann for her illuminating research.

I'm also profoundly grateful to the writers—living and gone—whose work is quoted or referenced in this book, whose words have been company, balm, and guide: W.H. Auden, Emily Dickinson, Joan Didion, John Donne, Andre Dubus, Louise Glück, Robert Hayden, Gerard Manley Hopkins, Fanny Howe, Rebecca Mead, John Milton, Flannery O'Connor, Cynthia Ozick, Emily Rapp Black, Adrienne Rich, Kevin Roose, Theodore Roethke, Mary Shelley, Natasha Trethewey, Richard Wilbur, and Christian Wiman.

I'm so lucky to have an incredible agent in Anna Stein, who helped this book come into being with patience, generosity, and remarkable clarity. Thank you for believing in it and in me.

My editor, Gabriel Fried, has been in the business of making my dreams come true from the moment I met him. Gabe, this book only exists because you dreamed it along with me, and I couldn't be more grateful for your intelligence, gentleness, friendship, and faith. Thank you for this version of my life.

Lucas Mann and Lauren Markham have continually championed and cheered on this project from afar, and their work has instructed, energized, and inspired me.

Laura Eve Engel, Helen Davies, Allison Serreas, Ashley Mullins, Jan Verberkmoes, Emily Rials, Heather McLeod, Molly Gail Shannon, and Taije Silverman: Your friendship and support mean everything. Thank you. I love you all.

To Alexandra Teague, who kept me company in one of the wildest years of my life, and whose feedback on this manuscript was astute, generous, and vital: inexpressible gratitude for your help and your friendship.

To Beth Ann Fennelly, to whom I owe every good thing, and whose insights on these essays were irreplaceable: Thank you for being my teacher, my champion, and my friend. You are a spectacular gift.

And to Susannah Nevison, who read every essay in this collection an uncountable number of times, whose insight, brilliance, and tenderness are threaded throughout it, and whose friendship is the force that made it possible: You know it all already. This book—like everything I've written, even before I knew it—is for you.

Finally, my family is the steadiest grace in the world. To Tim, Joanna, Kate, and Sarah; Helen and Bruce; Sheila, Craig, Julia, Eleanor, and Margot; Walker, Olivia, Kasandra, and Orion: all my love.

To my parents, Carrie and John Gregory: Being your daughter is the biggest stroke of luck I can imagine. I wouldn't trade a single piece of the life we've lived together. Thank you for all of it. For everything.

WORKS CITED

W. H. Auden, *Collected Poems* (New York: Modern Library, 2007).

Emily Dickinson, *The Complete Poems of Emily Dickinson*, ed. Thomas H. Johnson (New York : Little, Brown & Co., 1960).

Joan Didion, *Slouching Towards Bethlehem* (New York: Farrar, Straus & Giroux, 1968).

John Donne, *John Donne: The Major Works* (Oxford : Oxford University Press, 2009).

Andre Dubus, *Selected Stories* (Boston: David R. Godine Publishers, 1988).

T. S. Eliot, *Collected Poems 1909–1962* (London: Faber & Faber, 2002).

Louise Glück, *The Wild Iris* (New York: Ecco, 1992).

Judith E. Heumann, with Katherine Salinas and Michellie Hess, *Road Map for Inclusion: Changing the Face of Disability in Media* (https://www.fordfoundation.org/media/4276/judyheumann_report_2019_final.pdf).

Gerard Manley Hopkins, *Gerard Manley Hopkins: The Major Works* (Oxford: Oxford University Press, 2009).

Fanny Howe, "Theology and Poetry: an Interview with Fanny Howe," interviewed by Eve Grubin, *Lyric* (issue no. 7, 2005).

John Milton, *Paradise Lost*, ed. John Leonard (New York: Penguin, 2003).

Cynthia Ozick, *The Shawl* (New York: Knopf, 1989).

Adrienne Rich, *Diving into the Wreck* (New York: W. W. Norton & Co., 1973).

Theodore Roethke, *Collected Poems* (New York: Anchor, 1974).

Kevin Roose, *The Unlikely Disciple* (New York: Grand Central Publishing, 2009).

Emily Rapp Black, *Poster Child* (New York: Bloomsbury USA, 2006).

William Shakespeare, *Shakespeare's Sonnets*, ed. Katherine Duncan-Jones et al. (New York: The Arden Shakespeare, 2010).

Mary Shelley, *Frankenstein* (Oxford: Oxford University Press, 1994).

Natasha Trethewey, *Native Guard* (Boston: Houghton Mifflin, 2007).

Christian Wiman, *Every Riven Thing* (New York, Farrar, Straus & Girous, 2010).

James Wright, *Above the River: The Complete Poems and Selected Prose* (New York: Farrar, Straus & Giroux, 1990).

ABOUT THE AUTHOR

MOLLY MCCULLY BROWN is the author of the poetry collection *The Virginia State Colony for Epileptics and Feebleminded* (Persea Books, 2017), which won the 2016 Lexi Rudnitsky First Book Prize and was named a New York Times Critics' Top Book of 2017. With Susannah Nevison, she is also the coauthor of the poetry collection *In the Field Between Us*.

Brown has been the recipient of the Amy Lowell Poetry Traveling Scholarship, a United States Artists Fellowship, a Civitella Ranieri Foundation Fellowship, and the Jeff Baskin Writers Fellowship from the *Oxford American* magazine. Her poems and essays have appeared in *Tin House, Crazyhorse, The New York Times, Pleiades, Ninth Letter, Blackbird*, and elsewhere.

Raised in rural Virginia, she is a graduate of Bard College at Simon's Rock, Stanford University, and the University of Mississippi, where she received her MFA. She lives in Gambier, Ohio and teaches at Kenyon College, where she is the Kenyon Review Fellow in Poetry.